ABC of Eyes

Third edition

To our parents,
wives and children

ABC of Eyes

Third Edition

P T KHAW PhD FRCP FRCS FRCOphth
Professor and Consultant Ophthalmic Surgeon
Moorfields Eye Hospital and
Institute of Ophthalmology, University College London

A R ELKINGTON CBE FRCS FRCOphth
Professor of Ophthalmology
University of Southampton
Formerly President, Royal College of Ophthalmologists (1994–1997)

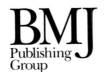
BMJ
Publishing
Group

© BMJ Books 1999
BMJ Books is an imprint of the BMJ Publishing Group

First published in 1988
by the BMJ Publishing Group, BMA House, Tavistock Square,
London WC1H 9JR

Second impression 1990
Third impression 1991
Fourth impression 1992
Fifth impression 1992
Sixth impression 1992
Seventh impression 1993
Eighth impression 1993
Second edition 1994
Second impression 1996
Third impression 1997
Fourth impression 1997
Fifth impression 1998
Third edition 1999

British Library Cataloguing in Publication Data

A catalogue record for this book is available
from the British Library

ISBN 0-7279-1262-3

Typeset by Apek Typesetters, Nailsea, Bristol
Printed in Singapore by Craft Print Pte Ltd

Contents

Acknowledgments

We would like to acknowledge the help we have received over the years from our general practitioner, medical student and ophthalmological colleagues; their probing questions have helped us to crystallise our thoughts on many topics. We are grateful to Alan Lacey from the Department of Medical Illustration at Moorfields Eye Hospital for his superb artistry and the diagrams. We would also like to thank Peggy Khaw for her tremendous work on the many drafts of the book from its inception, and Jennifer Murray and Suzy Couzens for their help with the 3rd edition. In the past Jane Smith, Mary Evans, Mary Banks, Deborah Reece and currently Alex Stibbe have also been very supportive, steering us through the pitfalls of publishing. We would also like to thank Stephen Tuft for his expert advice on the refractive surgery section. Jackie Martin, supported by the Royal London Society for the Blind, Barbara Norton and Jennifer Rignold guided us through the services for the visually handicapped. Finally we would like to thank Pharmacia Ltd for permission to use their colour plates on cataract surgery (page 29) and Guide Dogs for the Blind for the picture of the guide dog (page 44).

PTK
ARE
1999

1 History and examination

History

As in all clinical medicine, an accurate history and examination are essential if the correct diagnosis and treatment are to be achieved. Most ocular conditions can be diagnosed with a good history and simple examination techniques. Conversely, the failure to take a history and perform a simple examination can lead to conditions being missed that pose a threat to sight, or even to life.

The history may give many clues to the diagnosis. Visual symptoms are particularly important.

The rate of onset of visual symptoms gives an indication of the cause. A rapid deterioration in vision tends to be vascular in origin, whereas a gradual onset suggests a cause such as cataract. The loss of visual field may be characteristic, such as the central field loss of macular degeneration. Symptoms such as flashing lights may indicate traction on the retina and impending retinal detachment. Difficulties with work, reading, watching television and managing in the house should be identified. It is particularly important to assess the effect of the visual disability on the patient's lifestyle, especially as conditions such as cataract can, with modern techniques, be operated on at an early stage.

The patient should also be asked exactly what is worrying him as visual symptoms often cause great anxiety. Appropriate reassurance can then be given.

Questions about particular symptoms

Some specific questions are important in certain circumstances. If there has been ocular trauma, a history of any high velocity injury — particularly a hammer and chisel injury — should suggest an intraocular foreign body. Other questions, for example, about the type of discharge, may allow the diagnosis to be made in a patient with a red eye.

Ocular history — Easily forgotten, but essential. The patient's red eye may be associated with contact lens wear. A history of severe shortsightedness (myopia) considerably increases the risk of retinal detachment. Patients often forget to mention eye drops and eye operations if they are just asked about "drugs and operations". A purulent conjunctivitis requires much more urgent attention if the patient has previously had glaucoma drainage surgery, because of the risk of infection entering the eye.

Medical history — Many systemic disorders affect the eye, and the medical history may give clues to the cause of the problem; for instance, a vitreous haemorrhage in a patient with diabetes.

Family history —The best example of the importance of the family history is in the case of primary open angle glaucoma. This may be asymptomatic until severe visual damage has occurred. The risk of the disease may be up to 1:10 in first degree relatives, and the disease may be arrested if treated at an early stage. A family history of squint is also a risk factor for the development of squint.

Drug history — Many drugs affect the eye, and they should always be considered as a cause of ocular problems; for example, chloroquine may affect the retina.

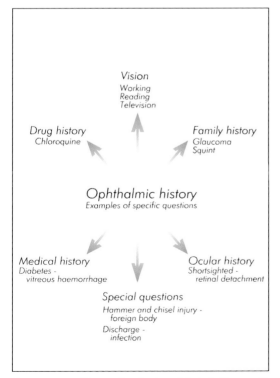

Vision
Working
Reading
Television

Drug history
Chloroquine

Family history
Glaucoma
Squint

Ophthalmic history
Examples of specific questions

Medical history
Diabetes -
vitreous haemorrhage

Ocular history
Shortsighted -
retinal detachment

Special questions
Hammer and chisel injury -
foreign body
Discharge -
infection

Answers to specific questions in the ophthalmic history will give clues to the diagnosis and help to exclude other problems.

Examination of the visual system

Assessment of vision.

- Snellen chart at 6 metres
- Snellen chart closer
- Counting fingers
- Hand movements
- Perception of light
- No perception of light

Vision

An assessment of visual acuity is fundamental in any ocular disorder, as it measures the function of the eye and gives some idea of the patient's disability. It may also have considerable medicolegal implications, as in the case of ocular damage at work or after assault.

Visual acuity is checked using a standard Snellen chart at 6 metres. If there is no room large enough a mirror can be used with a reversed Snellen chart at 3 metres. The numbers adjacent to the letters indicate the distance at which a person with no refractive error can read that line (hence the 6/60 line should normally be read at 60 metres). If the top line cannot be discerned the test can be done closer to the chart. If the chart cannot be read at 1 metre, patients may be asked to count fingers, and, if they cannot do that, to detect hand movements. Finally, it may be that they can perceive only light. From the patient's point of view, the functional difference between these categories may be the difference between managing at home on their own (count fingers) and total dependence on others (perception of light).

Vision should be tested with the aid of the patient's usual glasses or contact lenses. To achieve the optimal visual acuity, the patient should be asked to look through a pinhole. This reduces the effect of any refractive error. It is particularly useful if the patient cannot use contact lenses because of a red eye or has not brought his glasses. If patients cannot read English they can be asked to match letters; this is also useful for young children. Reading vision can be tested using a standard reading type book, or, if this is not available, various sizes of newspaper print. There may be quite a difference in the near and distance vision. A good example is presbyopia, which usually develops in the late forties owing to the failure of accommodation with age. Distance vision may be 6/6 without glasses but the patient may be able to read only larger newspaper print.

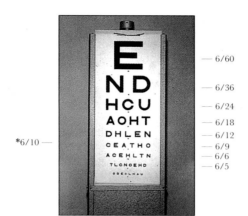

Testing visual acuity.

*Approximate level on Snellen chart required in at least one eye for driving a car

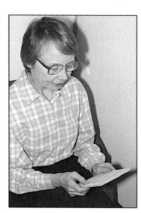

Testing reading vision.

Field of vision

Testing the visual field may give clues to the site of any lesion and the diagnosis.

Location of the lesion — Unilateral field loss in the lower nasal field suggests an upper temporal retinal lesion. Central field loss usually indicates macular problems. A homonymous hemianopia indicates problems in the brain rather than the eye, though the patient may present with visual disturbance.

Diagnosis — If the patient has a bitemporal field defect, this is most commonly caused by a pituitary tumour. A field defect arching over central vision to the blind spot (arcuate scotoma) is almost pathognomonic of glaucoma.

To test the visual field — the patient should be seated directly opposite the examiner and should then be asked to cover the eye that is not being tested and to look at the examiner's face. If there is a gross defect the patient will not be able to see part of the examiner's face and may be able to indicate this precisely: "I can't see the centre of your face".

If no gross defect is present the fields can be tested more formally. Testing the visual field using finger movements peripherally will show severe defects, but a more sensitive test is the detection of red colour, because the ability to detect red tends to be affected earlier. A red pin is

Testing visual fields

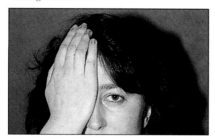

Ask patient to cover eye not being tested. Ensure that eye is completely covered by palm.

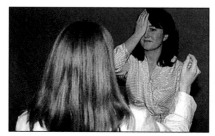

Move red pin in from periphery and ask patient to say when colour becomes apparent.

moved in from the periphery and the patient is asked when he can see something red. Finally, an extremely sensitive test is the comparison of the red in different quadrants. A good example is a patient who may have clinical signs of pituitary disease such as acromegaly; an early temporal defect can be detected if the patient is asked to compare the "quality" of the red colour in the upper temporal and nasal fields.

The pupils

Careful inspection of the pupils can show signs that are helpful in diagnosis. A bright torch is essential. A pupil stuck down to the lens is a result of inflammation within the eye, which is always serious. A peaked pupil after ocular injury suggests perforation with iris trapped in the wound. **Abnormal pupil reactions in the presence of ocular symptoms should always be treated seriously.**

The pupil's reactions to light are a simple way of checking the integrity of the visual pathways. By the time pupils do not react to direct light, however, the damage is very severe. A much more sensitive test is the relative difference in pupillary reactions. The torchlight is moved to and fro between the eyes not allowing time for the pupils to dilate. If one of the pupils does dilate when the light shines on it, there is a defect in the visual pathway on that side (relative afferent pupillary defect). Cataracts and macular degeneration do not usually cause an afferent pupillary defect unless the lesions are particularly advanced. Neurological disease must be suspected.

Other important and potentially life threatening conditions in which the pupils are affected include Horner's syndrome, where the pupil is small but reactive and there is an associated ptosis. This condition may be caused by an apical lung carcinoma. The well known Argyll Robertson pupils caused by syphilis (bilateral small irregular pupils with light-near dissociation) are rare. In a third nerve palsy there is ptosis and the eye is divergent. The pupil size and reactions in such a case give important clues to the aetiology. If the pupil is unaffected ("spared"), the cause is likely to be medical, e.g. diabetes or hypertension. If the pupil is dilated and fixed, the cause is probably surgical, e.g. a treatable intracranial aneurysm.

Eye position and movements

The appearance of the eyes shows the presence of any large degree of misalignment. This can, however, be misleading if the medial folds of the eyelid are wide. The position of the corneal reflections helps to confirm whether there is a true "squint". Squint and cover tests are dealt with in Chapter 10.

Patients should be asked if they have any double vision. If so, they should be asked to say whether diplopia occurs in any particular direction of gaze. It is important to exclude palsies of the third (eye turned out) or sixth (failure of abduction) cranial nerve, as these may be secondary to life threatening conditions. Complex abnormalities of eye movements should lead one to suspect myasthenia gravis or dysthyroid eye disease. The presence of nystagmus should be noted, as it may indicate significant neurological disease.

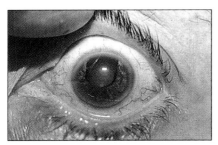

Torn peripheral iris (iridodialysis).

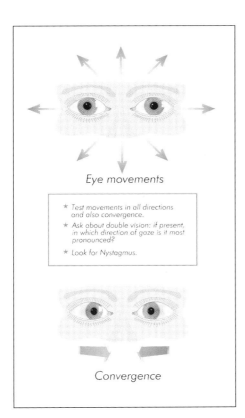

Distorted pupil after broad iridectomy.

Eye movements

★ Test movements in all directions and also convergence.

★ Ask about double vision: if present, in which direction of gaze is it most pronounced?

★ Look for Nystagmus.

Convergence

Test eye movements in all directions and when converging.

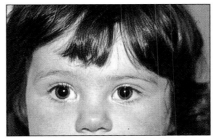

Normal position of corneal light reflexes.

History and examination

Eyelids Compare both sides and note position, lid lesions, and conditions of margins.

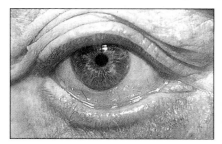

Ectropion.

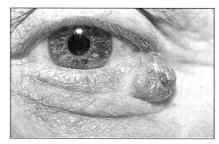

Basal cell carcinoma.

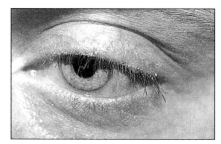

Blepharitis.

Conjunctiva and sclera
- Look for local or generalised inflammation
- Pull down lower lid and evert upper lid

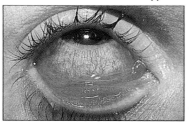

Conjunctivitis: generalised redness.

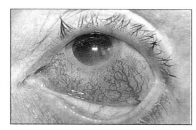

Scleritis: localised redness.

Cornea
- Look at clarity
- Stain with fluorescein

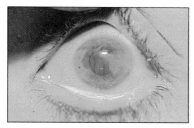

Corneal abrasion stained with fluorescein and illuminated with blue light.

Anterior chamber
- Check for blood and pus
- Check chamber depth

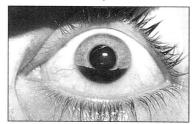

Blood in anterior chamber (hyphaema).

Optic disc, retina and macula

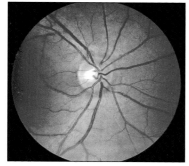

Normal optic disc.

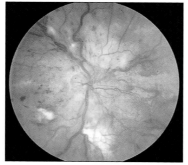

New vessels on optic disc in diabetes.

Eyelids, conjunctiva, sclera and cornea
Examination of the eyelids, conjunctiva, sclera, and cornea should be performed in good light and with magnification. The equipment needed is:
- a bright torch (with a blue filter for use with fluorescein);
- a magnifying aid;
- fluorescein impregnated strips or eye drops.

The lower lid should be pulled down to show the conjunctival lining and any secretions that may be in the lower fornix.

The cornea should then be stained with fluorescein eye drops; if this is not done many lesions, including large corneal ulcers, may be missed.

The anterior chamber should be examined, looking specifically at the depth, and for the presence of pus or blood.

If there are symptoms of "grittiness", a red eye or any history of foreign body the upper eyelid should be everted. This should not be done, however, if there is any question of ocular perforation as the ocular contents may prolapse.

Intraocular pressure
Assessment of intraocular pressure by palpation is useful only when the intraocular pressure is considerably raised, as in acute closed angle glaucoma. The eye should be gently palpated between two fingers and compared with the other eye or with the examiner's eye. The eye with acute glaucoma feels hard. Consider acute angle closure in any person over the age of 50 with a red eye.

Ophthalmoscopy
Good ophthalmoscopy is essential if many serious ocular and general diseases are not to be missed. To get a good view the pupil should be dilated. There is a risk of precipitating acute angle closure glaucoma, but this is very small. Patients should be warned to seek help immediately if they have symptoms of pain or haloes around lights after having their pupils dilated.

The best dilating drop is tropicamide 1%, which is short acting and has little effect on accommodation. The effects may still last several hours and the patient should be warned not to drive until any blurring of vision has subsided.

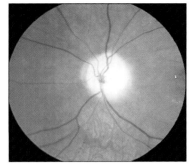

Optic atrophy.

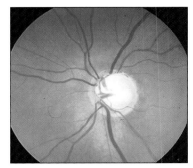

Glaucomatous cupping.

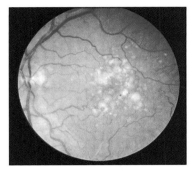

Age-related macular degeneration.

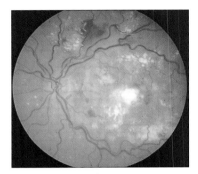

Diabetic maculopathy.

The ophthalmoscope should be set on the "0" lens. Patients should be asked to fix their gaze on an object in the distance as this reduces pupillary constriction and accomodation, and keeps the eye still. To enable a patient to fix on a distant object with the other eye, the examiner should use his right eye to examine the patient's right eye, and vice versa. The light should be shone at the eye until the red reflex is elicited. This red reflex is the reflection from the fundus. If this is absent or diminished there is an opacity between the cornea and retina. The commonest opacity is a cataract.

The optic disc should then be located and brought into focus with the lenses in the ophthalmoscope. If a patient has a high refractive error he can be asked to leave his glasses on, though this can cause more reflections. The physical signs at the disc may be the only chance of detecting serious disease in the patient. A blurred disc edge may be the only sign of a cerebral tumour. Cupping of the optic disc may be the only sign of undetected primary open angle glaucoma. New vessels at the disc may herald blinding proliferative retinopathy in a patient without symptoms. A pale disc may be the only stigma of past attacks of optic neuritis, or of a compressive cerebral tumour.

The retina should be scanned for abnormalities such as haemorrhages, exudates, or new vessels. The green filter on the ophthalmoscope helps to enhance blood vessels and microaneurysms. Finally the macula should be examined for the pigmentary changes of age-related macular degeneration and the exudates of diabetic maculopathy.

2 The red eye

The "red eye" is one of the most common ophthalmic problems presenting to the general practitioner. An accurate history is important and should pay particular attention to vision, degree and type of discomfort and the presence of a discharge. The history, and a good examination, will usually permit the diagnosis to be made without specialist ophthalmic equipment.

Symptoms and signs

The most important symptoms are pain and visual loss; these suggest serious conditions such as corneal ulceration, iritis and acute glaucoma. A purulent discharge suggests bacterial conjunctivitis; a clear discharge suggests a viral or allergic cause. A gritty sensation is common in conjunctivitis, but a foreign body must be excluded, particularly if only one eye is affected. **Corneal abrasions will be missed if fluorescein is not used.**

Equipment for an eye examination.

- Snellen eye chart
- Bright torch with blue filter
- Magnifying aid — for example, loupe
- Paper clip to help lid eversion
- Fluorescein impregnated strips or eye drops

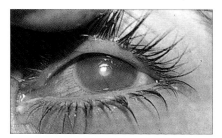

Corneal abscess (pseudomonas) in contact lens wearer.

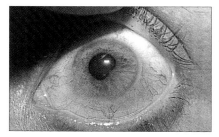

Anterior uveitis with ciliary flush around cornea and irregular stuck down pupil.

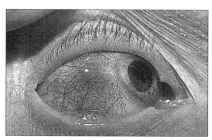

Scleritis.

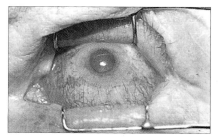

Acute angle closure glaucoma with red eye, semidilated pupil, and hazy cornea.

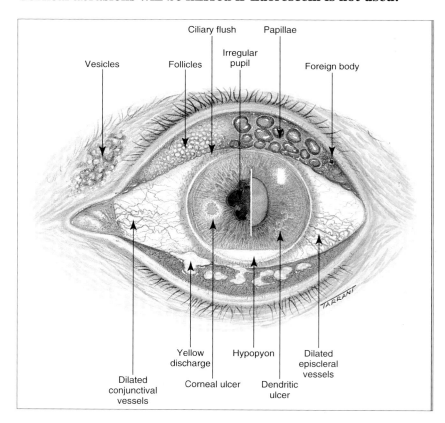

Important physical signs to look for in a patient with a red eye.

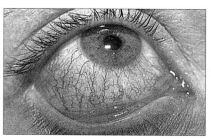

Bacterial conjunctivitis without discharge.

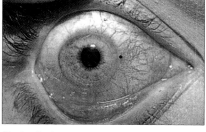

Foreign body.

Conjunctivitis

Conjunctivitis is one of the most common causes of an uncomfortable red eye. Conjunctivitis itself has many causes, including bacteria, viruses, chlamydia, and allergies.

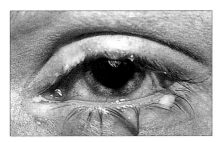
Adenovirus conjunctivitis of the right eye and enlarged preauricular nodes.

Bacterial conjunctivitis
History — The patient usually has discomfort and a purulent discharge in one eye that characteristically spreads to the other eye. The eye may be difficult to open in the morning because the discharge gums the lashes together. There may be a history of contact with a person with similar symptoms.

Examination — The vision should be normal after the discharge has been blinked clear of the cornea. The discharge is usually mucopurulent and there is uniform engorgement of all the conjunctival blood vessels. There is no staining of the cornea with fluorescein.

Management — Chloramphenicol eye drops should be instilled hourly for 24 hours, decreasing to four times a day for a week to hasten recovery. Chloramphenicol ointment applied at night may also increase comfort and reduce the morning eyelid stickiness. Patients should be advised about general hygiene measures; for example, not sharing face towels.

Viral conjunctivitis
Viral conjunctivitis is commonly associated with upper respiratory tract infections and is usually caused by an adenovirus. It is the type of conjunctivitis that occurs in epidemics.

History — The patient normally complains of both eyes being gritty and uncomfortable, although symptoms may begin in one eye. There may be associated symptoms of a cold and a cough. The discharge is usually watery. This type of conjunctivitis usually lasts longer than bacterial conjunctivitis and may go on for many weeks and patients need to be informed of this. Photophobia and discomfort may be severe if the patient goes on to develop discrete corneal opacities.

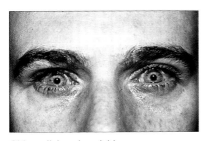
Purulent bacterial conjunctivitis.

Examination — Both eyes are red with diffuse conjunctival injection (engorged conjunctival vessels) and there may be a clear discharge. Small white lymphoid aggregations may be present on the conjunctiva (follicles). Small focal areas of corneal inflammation with erosions and associated opacities may give rise to pronounced symptoms, but these are difficult to see without high magnification. There may be associated head and neck lymphadenopathy.

Treatment — Viral conjunctivitis is generally a self-limiting condition, but chloramphenicol eye drops provide symptomatic relief and help prevent secondary bacterial infection. Viral conjunctivitis is extremely contagious and strict hygiene measures are important for both the patient and the doctor; for example, washing of hands and sterilising of instruments. In some patients the infection may have a chronic, protracted course and steroid eyedrops may be indicated if the corneal lesions and symptoms are persistent. **However, steroids must not be prescribed without ophthalmological supervision. Furthermore, if long term steroids are required, patients should remain under continuous ophthalmological supervision.**

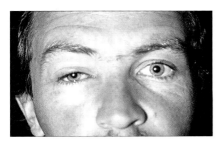
Viral conjunctivitis.

Chlamydial conjunctivitis
History — Patients are usually young with a history of a chronic bilateral conjunctivitis with a mucopurulent discharge. There may be associated symptoms of venereal disease.

Examination — There is bilateral diffuse conjunctival injection with a mucopurulent discharge. There are many lymphoid aggregates in the conjunctiva (follicles). The cornea is usually involved (keratitis) and an infiltrate of the upper cornea (pannus) may be seen.

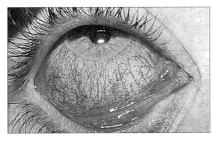
Chlamydial conjunctivitis.

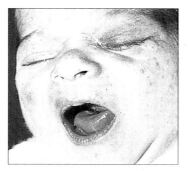

Infantile conjunctivitis.

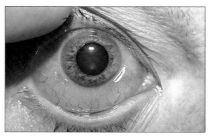

Chemosis: pollen allergy.

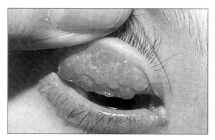

Large papillae in allergic conjunctivitis.

> **Topical steroids should not be prescribed or continued without continuous ophthalmological supervision**

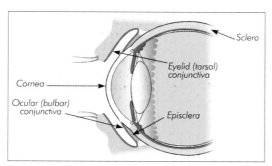

Conjunctiva, sclera, and episclera.

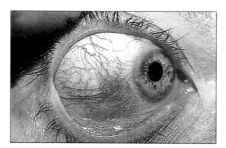

Episcleritis.

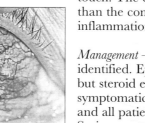

Scleritis.

Management — The diagnosis is often difficult and special bacteriological tests may be necessary to confirm the clinical suspicions. Treatment comprises tetracycline ointment and oral tetracyline 250 mg four times a day for at least a month. Associated venereal disease should also be treated. Worldwide, trachoma is one of the major causes of blindness. In developing countries infection by *Chlamydia trachomatis* results in severe scarring of the conjunctiva and the underlying tarsal plate. The eyelids turn in and permanently scar the already damaged cornea.

Conjunctivitis in infants
Conjunctivitis in young children is extremely important because the eye defences are immature and a severe conjunctivitis with membrane formation and bleeding may occur. Serious corneal disease and blindness may result. **Conjunctivitis in an infant less than one month old (ophthalmia neonatorum) is a notifiable disease.** Such babies must be seen in an eye department so that special cultures can be taken and appropriate treatment given. Venereal disease in the parents must be excluded.

Allergic conjunctivitis
History — The main feature of allergic conjunctivitis is itching. Both eyes are usually affected and there may be a clear discharge. There may be a family history of atopy or recent contact with chemicals or eye drops. Similar symptoms may have occurred at the same time in previous years.

Examination — The conjunctivae are diffusely injected and may be oedematous (chemosis). The discharge is clear and stringy. Because of the fibrous septa that tether the eyelid (tarsal) conjunctivae, oedema results in round swellings (papillae). When these are large they are referred to as cobblestones.

Treatment — Topical antihistamine and vasoconstrictor eye drops provide short term relief. Eye drops which prevent degranulation of mast cells are also useful but they may need to be used for several weeks to achieve maximal effect. Oral antihistamines may also be used, particularly the newer compounds which cause less sedation. Topical steroids are effective, but should not be used without regular ophthalmological supervision because of the risk of steroid-induced cataracts and glaucoma, which may irreversibly damage vision.

Episcleritis and scleritis

Episcleritis and scleritis usually present as a localised area of inflammation. The episclera lies just beneath the conjunctiva and adjacent to the tough white scleral coat of the eye. Both the sclera and episclera may become inflamed, particularly in rheumatoid arthritis and other autoimmune conditions, but no cause is found for most cases of episcleritis.

History — The patient complains of a red and sore eye that may also be tender. There may be reflex lacrimation but usually there is no discharge. Scleritis is much more painful than episcleritis.

Examination — There is a localised area of inflammation that is tender to touch. The episcleral and scleral vessels are larger than the conjunctival vessels. The signs of inflammation are usually more florid in scleritis.

Management — Any underlying cause should be identified. Episcleritis is essentially self limiting, but steroid eye drops hasten recovery and provide symptomatic relief. Scleritis is much more serious, and all patients need ophthalmological review. Serious systemic disorders need to be excluded, and systemic immunosuppressive treatment may be required.

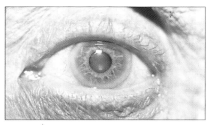

Eye with herpes simplex ulcer (not visible without fluorescein).

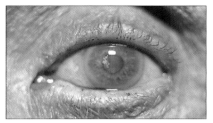

Same eye stained with fluorescein and viewed with blue light (ulcer visible).

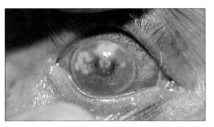

Herpes simplex ulcers inadvertently treated with steroids. Ulceration has spread and deepened.

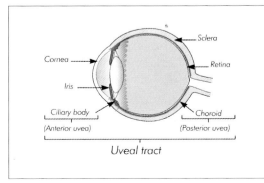

Corneal abscess with pus in anterior chamber (hypopyon).

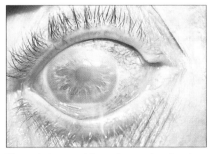

Different parts of the eye that may be affected by uveitis.

Corneal ulceration

Corneal ulcers may be caused by bacterial, viral, and fungal infections; these may occur as primary events or may be secondary to an event that has compromised the eye — for example, abrasion, contact lens wear, or use of topical steroids.

History — Pain is usually a prominent feature as the cornea is an exquisitely sensitive organ, though this is not so when corneal sensation is impaired; for example, after herpes zoster ophthalmicus. Indeed, this lack of sensation may be the cause of the ulceration. There may be clues such as similar past attacks, facial cold sores, a recent abrasion, or the wearing of contact lenses.

Examination — Visual acuity depends on the location and size of the ulcer, and normal visual acuity does not exclude an ulcer. There may be a watery discharge due to reflex lacrimation or a mucopurulent discharge in bacterial ulcers. Conjunctival injection may be generalised or localised if the ulcer is peripheral, giving a clue to its presence. Fluorescein must be used or an ulcer may easily be missed. Certain types of corneal ulceration are characteristic. If there is inflammation in the anterior chamber there may be a collection of pus present (hypopyon). The upper eyelid must be everted or a subtarsal foreign body causing corneal ulceration may be missed. Patients with subtarsal foreign bodies sometimes do not recollect anything entering the eye.

Management — Patients with corneal ulceration should be referred urgently to an eye department or the eye may be lost. Management depends on the cause of the ulceration. The diagnosis may usually be made on the clinical appearance. The appropriate swabs and cultures should be arranged to try to identify the causative organism. Intensive treatment is then started with drops and ointment of broad spectrum antibiotics until the organisms and their sensitivities to various antibiotics are known. Injections of antibiotics into the subconjunctival space may be given to increase local concentrations of the drugs. Cycloplegic drops are used to relieve pain resulting from spasm of the ciliary muscle, and as they are also mydriatics they prevent adhesions of the iris to the lens (posterior synechiae). Systemic steroids may be used to reduce local inflammatory damage not caused by direct infection, but the indications for their use are specific and they should not be used without ophthalmological supervision.

Iritis, iridocyclitis, and anterior uveitis

The iris, ciliary body and choroid are embryologically similar and are known as the uveal tract. Inflammation of the iris (iritis) does not occur without inflammation of the ciliary body (cyclitis) and together these are referred to as iridocyclitis, or anterior uveitis. Thus the terms are synonymous.

Several groups of patients are at risk, including those who have had past attacks of iritis, and those with a seronegative arthropathy, particularly if they are positive for the HLA B27 histocompatibility antigen; for example, a young man with ankylosing spondylitis. Children with seronegative arthritis are also at high risk, particularly if they have only a few joints affected by the arthritis.

The uveitis in these conditions may be relatively asymptomatic and they may suffer serious ocular damage if they are not screened. Sarcoidosis also causes chronic anterior uveitis, as do several other conditions including herpes zoster ophthalmicus, syphilis and tuberculosis.

History — The patient who has had past attacks can often feel an attack coming on even before physical signs are present. There is often pain in the later stages with photophobia due to inflammation and ciliary spasm. The pain may be worse when the patient is reading and contracting his ciliary muscle.

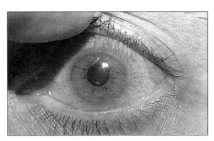

Anterior uveitis/iritis with ciliary flush but pupil not stuck down.

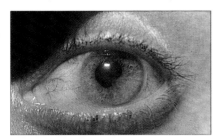

Anterior uveitis with ciliary flush and irregular pupil.

Examination — The vision may initially be normal but later it may be impaired. Accommodation, and hence reading vision, may be affected. There may be inflammatory cells in the anterior chamber, cataracts may form and adhesions may develop between the iris and lens. The affected eye is red with the injection being particularly pronounced over the area covering the inflamed ciliary body (ciliary flush). The pupil is small because of spasm of the sphincter or irregular because of adhesions of the iris to the lens (posterior synechiae). An abnormal pupil in a red eye usually indicates serious ocular disease. Inflammatory cells may be deposited on the back of the cornea (keratitic precipitates) or may settle to form a collection of cells in the anterior chamber of the eye (hypopyon).

Management — If there is an underlying cause it must be treated, but in many cases no cause is found. It is important to ensure there is no disease in the rest of the eye that is giving rise to signs of an anterior uveitis such as more posterior inflammation, a retinal detachment or an intraocular tumour. Treatment is with topical steroids to reduce the inflammation and prevent adhesions within the eye. The ciliary body is paralysed to relieve pain, and the associated dilation of the pupil also prevents the development of adhesions between the iris and lens that can cause "pupil block" glaucoma. The intraocular pressure may also rise because inflammatory cells block the trabecular meshwork and antiglaucoma treatment may have to be given if this occurs. Continued inflammation may lead to permanent damage of the trabecular meshwork and secondary glaucoma, cataracts, and oedema of the macula.

Acute angle closure glaucoma

Acute glaucoma should always be considered in a patient over the age of 50 with a painful red eye. The diagnosis must not be missed or the eye will be permanently damaged. The mechanism is dealt with in Chapter 8.

History — The attack usually comes on quite quickly, characteristically in the evening, when the pupil becomes semidilated. There is pain in one eye, which can be extremely severe and may be accompanied by vomiting. The patient complains of impaired vision and haloes around lights due to oedema of the cornea. The patient may have had similar attacks in the past which were relieved by going to sleep (the pupil constricts during sleep, so relieving the attack).

Examination — The eye is inflamed and tender. The cornea is hazy and the pupil is semidilated and fixed. Vision is impaired according to the state of the cornea. On gentle palpation the eye feels harder than the other eye. The anterior chamber seems shallower than usual, with the iris being close to the cornea. If the patient is seen after the resolution of an attack the signs may have disappeared, hence the importance of the history.

Management — Urgent referral to hospital is required. Emergency treatment is needed if the sight in the eye is to be preserved. If it is not possible to get the patient to hospital straight away, intravenous acetazolamide (Diamox) 500 mg should be given, and pilocarpine 4% should be instilled in the eye to constrict the pupil. The pressure must first be brought down medically and a hole then made in the iris with a laser (iridotomy) or surgically (iridectomy) to restore normal aqueous flow. The other eye should be treated prophylactically in a similar way. If treatment is delayed adhesions may form between the iris and the cornea (peripheral anterior synechiae) or the trabecular meshwork may be irreversibly damaged necessitating a full surgical drainage procedure.

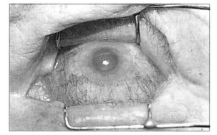

Acute angle closure glaucoma. Note the corneal oedema (irregular reflected image of light on cornea) and fixed semi-dilated pupil.

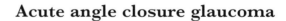

Features of acute angle closure glaucoma.

● Pain	● Hazy cornea
● Haloes round lights	● Age more than 50
● Impaired vision	● Eye feels hard
● Fixed semidilated pupil	● Unilateral

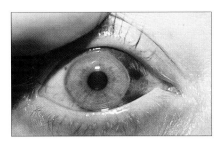

Subconjunctival haemorrhage.

Subconjunctival haemorrhage

History — The patient usually presents with a red eye which is comfortable and without any visual disturbance. It is usually the appearance of the eye that has made the patient seek attention. If there is a history of trauma, or a red eye after hammering or chiseling, then ocular injury and an intraocular foreign body must be excluded.

Examination — There is a localised area of subconjunctival blood which is usually relatively well demarcated. There is no discharge or conjunctival reaction.

Management — It is worth checking the blood pressure to exclude hypertension. If there are no other abnormalities the patient should be reassured and told the redness may take several weeks to fade.

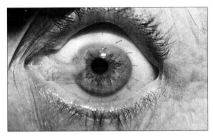

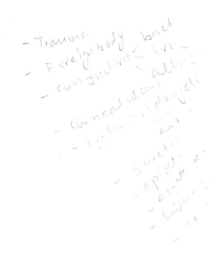

Pterygium.

Inflamed pterygium or pinguecula

History — The patient complains of a focal localised red area or lump in the interpalpebral area. There may have been a pre-existing lesion in the area that patients may have noticed before.

Examination — Pingueculae are degenerative areas on the conjunctiva found in the 4 and 8 o'clock positions adjacent to, but not invading, the cornea. These common lesions may be related to sun and wind exposure. Occasionally they become inflamed or ulcerated. A pterygium is a non-malignant fibrovascular growth that encroaches onto the cornea, and probably related to exposure.

Treatment — If the pinguecula is ulcerated antibiotics may be indicated. For a pterygium, surgical excision is indicated if it is a cosmetic problem, causes irritation or is encroaching on the visual axis.

3 Eyelid and lacrimal disorders

Lumps in the lid

The most common lump found in the eyelid is a chalazion, but the accurate diagnosis of a lid lump is important because the lump:

- *may necessitate a disfiguring operation if not treated early* — basal cell carcinoma;
- *may be life threatening* — a deep invading basal cell carcinoma;
- *may be the cause of visual disturbance* — a chalazion pressing on the cornea and causing astigmatism;
- *may indicate systemic disease* — xanthelasmas in a patient with hyperlipidaemia;
- *may cause amblyopia* — if it obstructs vision in a young child.

Chalazion
A chalazion (meibomian cyst) is a granuloma of the lipid-secreting meibomian glands that lie in the lid. It is probably the result of a blocked duct with local reaction to the accumulation of lipid.

The patient may initially complain of a lump in the lid that is hard and inflamed. This settles and the patient is left with a discrete lump in the lid that may cause astigmatism and consequent blurring of vision. Clinically there is a hard lump in the lid, which is clearly visible when the lid is everted.

Many chalazia settle on conservative treatment. This comprises warm compresses (with a towel soaked in warm water) and the application of chloramphenicol ointment. If the chalazion is uncomfortable, excessively large, persistent, or disturbing vision it can be incised and curetted under local anaesthesia from the inner conjunctival side of the eyelid.

Recurrent chalazia may suggest an underlying problem such as blepharitis, a skin disorder such as acne rosacea, or very rarely even a malignant tumour of the meibomian glands.

Stye
A stye and chalazion are often confused. A stye is an infection of a lash follicle, causing a red, tender swelling at the lid margin. Unlike a chalazion, a stye may have a "head" of pus at the lid margin. It should be treated with warm compresses to help it to discharge, and chloramphenicol ointment should be used.

Marginal cysts
Marginal cysts may develop from the lipid- and sweat-secreting glands round the margins of the eyelids. They are dome shaped with no inflammation. The cysts of the sweat glands are filled with clear fluid (cyst of Moll) and the cysts of the lipid secreting glands are filled with yellowish contents (cyst of Zeiss).

Importance of lumps in the eyelid.

- May need disfiguring operations if left
- May be life threatening
- May be the cause of visual disturbance
- May cause blindness in children
- May indicate systemic disease

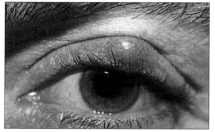

Chalazion.

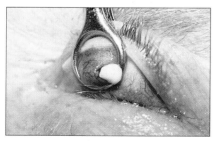

Incised chalazion.

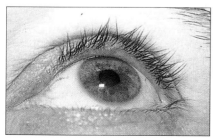

Stye.

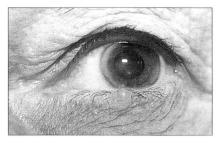

Cyst of sweat secreting gland (cyst of Moll).

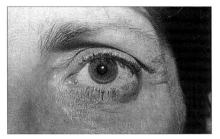

Xanthelasmas and corneal arcus in a young patient.

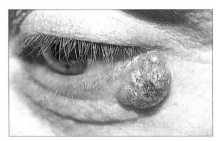

Basal cell carcinoma.

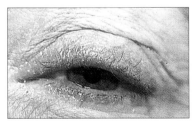

Blepharitis.

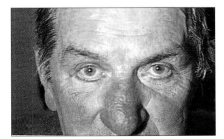

Rosacea with associated blepharitis.

No treatment is indicated for marginal cysts causing no problems. If they are a cosmetic blemish they can be removed under local anaesthesia.

Papilloma
Papillomas are often pedunculated and multilobular. They are common and may be caused by viruses. They should be removed if they are large and the diagnosis is uncertain, or if they are disfiguring.

Xanthelasma
Xanthelasmas may be an incidental finding, or the patient may complain of yellow plaques on the nasal sides of the eyelids; these contain lipid. Associated hyperlipidaemia must be excluded and the lesions may be removed under local anaesthesia if they cause a cosmetic problem.

Basal cell carcinoma
Basal cell carcinoma (rodent ulcer) is the most common malignant tumour of the eyelid. It occurs mainly in the lower lid, which is particularly exposed to sunlight. The tumour does not metastasise, but may be life threatening if allowed to infiltrate locally. If it is large when the patient is referred, an extensive and often disfiguring operation may be necessary.

The classical basal cell carcinoma has a pearly rounded edge with a necrotic centre, but it may be difficult to diagnose if it presents as a diffuse indurated lesion. It is particularly easy to miss the invasive form that occurs in a skin crease, which may be invading deeply with few cutaneous signs.

The patient should be referred urgently if there is any suspicion of a basal cell carcinoma. It is usually excised under local anaesthesia, unless complicated plastic surgery is required. Radiotherapy may also be used.

Inflammatory disease of the eyelid

Blepharitis
Blepharitis is a common condition but is often not diagnosed. It is a chronic disease; the patient complains of persistently sore eyes. The symptoms may be intermittent and include a gritty sensation and sore eyelids. The patient may present with a chalazion or stye, which are much more common in patients with blepharitis, and these may be recurrent. Physical signs include inflamed lid margins, blocked meibomian gland orifices, and crusts round the lid margins. The conjunctiva may be inflamed, and punctate staining of the cornea may be visible on staining with fluorescein. Associated skin diseases include rosacea, eczema, and psoriasis. The aims of treatment are to:

- *keep the lids clean* — the crusts and coagulated lipid should be gently cleaned with a cotton wool bud dipped in warm water. This can be combined with baby shampoo to help remove lipid;

- *treat infection* — antibiotic ointment should be smeared on the lid margin to help kill the staphylococci in the lid that may be aggravating the condition. This may be done for several months;

- *replace tears* — the tear film in patients with blepharitis is abnormal, and artificial tears may provide considerable relief of symptoms;

- *treat sebaceous gland dysfunction* — in severe cases, or those associated with sebaceous gland dysfunction, such as rosacea, oral tetracycline may be invaluable. Indications for referral are poor response to treatment and corneal disease.

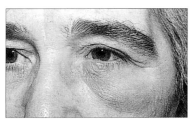

Chalazion with associated inflammation of lower eyelid.

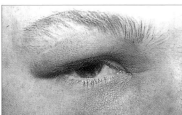

Inflammation of upper eyelid after expression of blackhead.

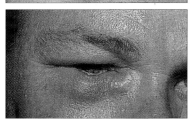

Dacryocystitis.

Orbital cellulitis can cause blindness if not treated immediately — particularly in children

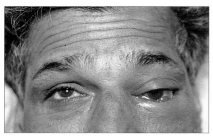

Orbital cellulitis: swollen eyelids, conjunctival swelling, displaced eyeball, and restricted eye movements.

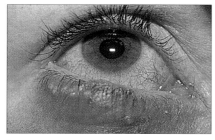

Herpes simplex with associated conjunctivitis.

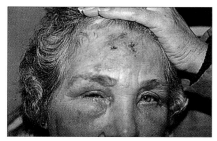

Herpes zoster ophthalmicus with swollen eyelids.

Acute inflammation of the eyelid

It is important to achieve a diagnosis in a patient with an acutely inflamed eyelid as some conditions may be blinding — for example, orbital cellulitis. There are several causes.

A chalazion or stye — Routine treatment should be given for these conditions. In addition, if infection is spreading, systemic antibiotics may be indicated.

Spread of local infection — Infection may have spread from a local lesion such as a "squeezed" comedo. Again, if there is spread of infection, systemic antibiotics are indicated.

Acute dacryocystitis — In this condition, the site of inflammation is medial, over the lacrimal sac. There may be a history of previous watering of the eye as a result of a blocked lacrimal system that has since become infected. Treatment is with topical chloramphenicol and systemic antibiotics until the infection resolves. Recurrent attacks of dacryocystitis or symptomatic watering of the eye are indications for operation.

Orbital cellulitis — **This is a potentially blinding and life threatening condition and must not be missed.** Orbital cellulitis usually results from the spread of infection from adjacent sinuses. It is particularly important in children, in whom blindness can ensue within hours.

The patient usually presents with unilateral swollen eyelids that may or may not be red. Features to look for include:
● the patient is unwell;
● there is tenderness over the sinuses;
● there is restriction of eye movements.

The possibility of orbital cellulitis should always be kept in mind, especially in children, and patients should be referred immediately.

Allergy — There may be a history of contact with an allergen, including animals, plants, chemicals or cosmetics. Itching is a good indicator of allergy and the allergen should be avoided. Treatment may include the application of a weak topical steroid ointment; for example, hydrocortisone 1% onto the eyelid for a short period.

Herpes simplex — May present as a vesicular rash on the skin of the eyelid. There may be associated areas of vesicular eruption on the face. An "experienced" patient may be able to discern the prodromal tingling sensation. Early application of aciclovir cream will shorten the length and severity of the episode. Associated ocular herpetic disease should be considered if the eye is red, and the patient should then be referred immediately.

Herpes zoster ophthalmicus (shingles) — Presents as a vesicular rash over the distribution of the ophthalmic division of the fifth cranial nerve. There may be associated pain and the patient usually feels unwell.

The eye is often affected, particularly if the side of the nose is also affected (which is innervated by a branch of the nasociliary nerve that also innervates the eye). Common ocular problems include conjunctivitis, keratitis, and uveitis. The eye is often shut because of oedema of the eyelid, but an attempt should be made to inspect the globe. If the eye is red or if there is visual disturbance the patient should be referred straight away. The ocular complications of herpes zoster may occur late in the disease, so the eye should be examined at each visit.

Treatment includes application of a wetting cream to the skin after crusting, to prevent painful and disfiguring scars. If the eye is affected, topical antibiotics may prevent secondary infection, and aciclovir ointment is used. Oral aciclovir given early in the course of the disease may reduce the incidence of long term sequelae such as pain.

Malpositions of the eyelids and eyelashes

Malpositions of the eyelids and eyelashes are common and give rise to various symptoms, including irritation of the eye by lashes rubbing on it (entropion and ingrowing eyelashes) and watering of the eye caused by malposition of the punctum (ectropion).

The eyelids are folds of skin with fibrous plates in both the upper and lower lids, and the circular muscle (orbicularis) controls the closing of the eye. Any change in the muscles or supporting tissues may result in malposition of the lids.

Entropion
The patient may present complaining of irritation caused by eyelashes rubbing on the cornea. This may be immediately apparent on examination but may be intermittent, in which case the lid may be in the normal position.The clue is that the eyelashes of the lower lid are pushed to the side by the regular inturning, and the cornea should be examined by staining with fluorescein. The entropion can be brought on by asking the patient to close their eyes tightly, and then open the eyes. Entropion is common, particularly in elderly patients with some spasm of the eyelids. The great danger of entropion is ulceration and scarring of the cornea by the abrading eyelashes.

Temporary treatment of entropion consists of taping down the lower lid and applying chloramphenicol ointment. An operation under local anaesthesia is required to permanently correct the entropion. Scarring of the cornea associated with entropion resulting from trachoma is one of the commonest causes of blindness worldwide.

Trichiasis
Sometimes the lid may be in a normal position, but aberrant eyelashes may grow inwards. Trichiasis is more common in the presence of diseases of the eyelid such as blepharitis or trachoma. The eyelashes can be seen on examination, especially with magnification. They can be pulled out, but they frequently regrow. The application of chloramphenicol ointment helps to prevent corneal damage, and electrolysis of the hair roots or cryotherapy may be necessary to stop the lashes regrowing.

Ectropion
The initial complaint may be that of a watery eye. The tears drain mainly via the lower punctum at the medial end of the lower lid. If the eyelid is not properly apposed to the eye, tears cannot flow into the punctum and the result is a watery eye. The patient may also complain of the unsightly appearance of an ectropion. The most common reason for ectropion is laxity of tissues of the lid as a result of ageing, but it also occurs if the muscles are weak, as in the case of a facial nerve palsy. Scarring of the skin of the eyelid may also pull the lid margin down.

Ectropion can be rectified by an operation under local anaesthesia. The use of ointment before the operation will help to protect the eye and prevent drying of the exposed conjunctiva.

Ptosis
Ptosis or drooping of the eyelid may:
- *indicate a life threatening condition* — such as a third nerve palsy secondary to aneurysm, or a Horner's syndrome secondary to carcinoma of the lung;
- *indicate a disease that needs systemic treatment* — such as myasthenia gravis;
- *cause irreversible amblyopia in a child* as a result of the lid obstructing vision. If there is any question of a ptosis obstructing vision in a child, he or she should be urgently referred;
- *be easily treatable by a simple operation* — as in senile ptosis.

Main symptoms of lid and lash malposition.

- Irritation of the eye by lashes rubbing on it (entropion)
- Watering of the eye caused by malposition of the punctum (ectropion)

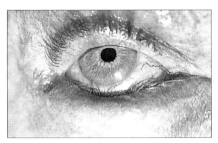

Entropion. Inturning eyelashes may scratch and damage the cornea.

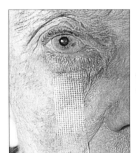

Temporary treatment of entropion.

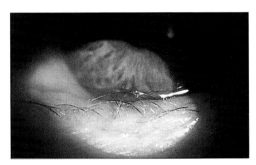

Trichiasis.

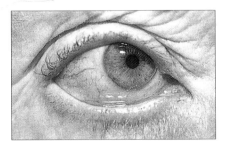

Ectropion with resulting epiphora.

Ptosis may occasionally:

- Indicate a life threatening disease
- Indicate a systemic disease
- Cause amblyopia in children

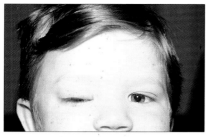

Ptosis caused by lid haemangioma: exclude amblyopia in a child.

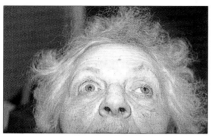

Left ptosis caused by pupil sparing third nerve palsy: note the divergent eye.

The patient will usually complain of a drooping eyelid. The upper eyelid is raised by the levator muscle, which is controlled by the third nerve. There is also Müller's muscle, which is controlled by the sympathetic nervous system. These muscles are attached to the fibrous plate in the eyelid and other lid structures. The ptosis can occur because of defects in the following tissues:

Lid tissues — With ageing the tissues of the eyelid become lax and the connections loosen resulting in ptosis; this is common in the elderly. The eye movements and pupils should be normal. A pseudoptosis may occur when the eyelid skin sags and droops down over the lid margin. Both these conditions are amenable to relatively simple operations under local anaesthesia.

Muscle tissue — It is important not to miss a general muscular disorder such as myasthenia gravis or dystrophia myotonica in a patient presenting with ptosis. Any diplopia, worsening symptoms throughout the day, and other muscular symptoms should lead one to suspect myasthenia. The patient's facies and handshake may give clues to the diagnosis of dystrophia myotonica.

Nerve supply — A third nerve palsy may present as a ptosis. This together with an abducted eye and dilated pupil, indicates the diagnosis. The patient should be urgently referred as causes of third nerve palsy include a compressive lesion of the third nerve such as an aneurysm. Diabetes should be excluded.

Horner's syndrome resulting from damage to the sympathetic chain — The pupil will be small but reactive, and sweating over the affected side of the face may be reduced. The eye movements should be normal. Causes of Horner's syndrome include lesions of the brain stem and spinal cord, and apical lung tumours, so the patient should be referred.

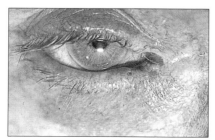

Normal tear flow.

The lacrimal system

The watering eye
Tears are produced by the lacrimal glands that lie in the upper lateral aspect of the orbit. They flow down across the eye along the lid margins and are spread across the eye by blinking. They then flow through the upper and lower puncta to the lacrimal sac and down the nasolacrimal duct into the nose. A watering eye may occur for several reasons.

Excessive production of tears — This is rare, but can occur paradoxically in a patient with "dry eyes". Basal secretion of tears is inadequate and this results in drying of the eye. This gives rise to a reactive secretion of tears that causes epiphora. The patient may give a history of intermittent discomfort followed by watering of the eye.

Punctal malposition secondary to lid malposition — The puncta must be well apposed to the eye to drain tears. Even mild ectropion can result in pooling of tears and overflow. Careful examination of the lid will usually show any malposition, which may be remedied by performing a minor operation.

Punctal stenosis — The puncta may close up and this will result in watering. If this is the case, the puncta cannot be seen easily on examination with a magnifying loupe. They can be surgically dilated or opened by a minor operation under local anaesthesia.

Blockage of the lacrimal sac or nasolacrimal duct — If the nasolacrimal duct is blocked and cannot be freed by syringing, an operation may be required. A common operation to bypass the obstruction is a dacryocystorhinostomy

Watering eye caused by punctal ectropion.

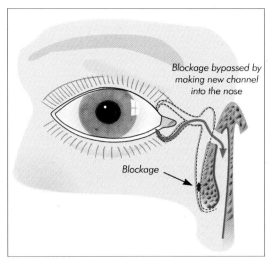

Dacryocystorhinostomy (DCR).

(DCR), in which a hole is made through into the nose from the lacrimal sac. Sometimes plastic tubes are left in for several months to create a fistula. This major operation is usually performed under general anaesthesia.

In children the lacrimal drainage system may not be patent, particularly in the first few years of life. The child will present with a watering eye, or sometimes with recurrent conjunctivitis. Treatment is usually with chloramphenicol eye drops for episodes of conjunctivitis, and

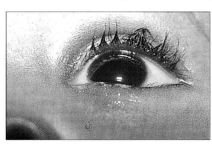

Blocked left nasolacrimal system in a child with recurrent discharge.

the parents should be advised to massage the lacrimal sac daily to encourage flow. Most cases in childhood will resolve spontaneously. If the watering persists, the child may have to have the sac and duct probed under general anaesthesia. If the blockage persists a dacryocystorhinostomy may be performed when the child is older, but this is not often necessary.

The dry eye

The dry eye is common in the elderly in whom tear secretion is reduced. The patient usually presents complaining of a chronic gritty sensation in the eye which is not particularly red. Systemic diseases such as rheumatoid arthritis are associated with a dry eye. Drugs such as diuretics may also exacerbate the symptoms of a dry eye. Staining of the cornea may be apparent with fluorescein and rose bengal eye drops. If rose bengal eye drops are used, the eyes must be washed out very thoroughly as these drops are a potent irritant. Treatment includes:

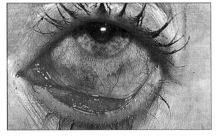

Dry eye in rheumatoid arthritis, stained with rose bengal drops which stain damaged epithelium.

- artificial tear drops, which may be used as frequently as necessary;
- simple ointment, which helps to give prolonged lubrication, particularly at night when tear secretion is minimal;
- acetylcysteine eye drops, which are useful if there is clumping of mucus on the eye (filamentary keratitis). However many patients find that the drops sting;
- treatment of any associated blepharitis.

4 Injuries to the eye

An injury to the eye or its surrounding tissues is the most common cause for attendance at an eye hospital accident and emergency department.

History

The history of how the injury was sustained is crucial, as it gives clues to what to look for during the examination. **If there is a history of any high velocity injury (particularly a hammer and chisel injury) a penetrating injury must be strongly suspected and excluded.** If there has been a forceful blunt injury (such as a punch), signs of a "blow out" fracture should be sought. The circumstances of the injury must be elicited and carefully recorded as these may have important medicolegal implications.

Examination

A good examination is vital if there is history of eye injury. Specific signs must be looked for or they will be missed. These are illustrated below. It is vital to test visual acuity both to establish a baseline value and to alert the examiner to the possibility of further problems, although an acuity of 6/6 does not necessarily exclude serious problems — even a penetrating injury. The visual acuity may also have considerable medicolegal implications. Local anaesthetic may need to be used to obtain a good view, and the use of fluorescein is mandatory if an abrasion is not to be missed.

Common types of eye injury.

- Corneal abrasions
- Foreign bodies
- Radiation damage
- Chemical damage
- Blunt injuries
- Penetrating injuries

The injured eye.

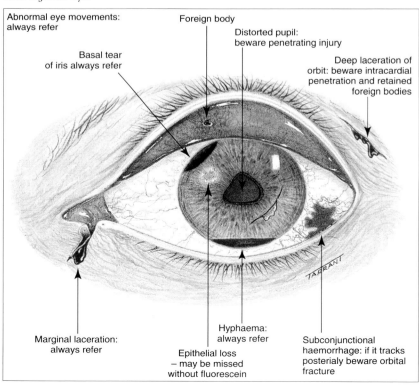

Abnormal eye movements: always refer

Foreign body

Distorted pupil: beware penetrating injury

Basal tear of iris always refer

Deep laceration of orbit: beware intracardial penetration and retained foreign bodies

Marginal laceration: always refer

Epithelial loss – may be missed without fluorescein

Hyphaema: always refer

Subconjunctional haemorrhage: if it tracks posterialy beware orbital fracture

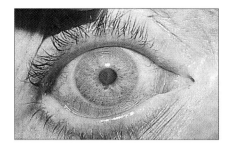

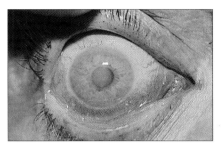

Corneal abrasion stained with fluorescein and illuminated with white light (top) and blue light (above).

Corneal abrasions

Corneal abrasions are the most common result of blunt injury. They may follow injuries with foreign bodies, fingernails or twigs. **Abrasions will be missed if fluorescein is not instilled.**

The aims of treatment are:
- *to speed healing and protect the eye* — pad the eye;
- *to prevent infection* — apply chloramphenicol ointment;
- *to relieve pain* — instil a cycloplegic (homatropine 2%); give oral analgesia if necessary.

The drops will relieve ciliary spasm and dilate the pupil. The patient uses an eye pad for a day or so until the abrasion heals and the chloramphenicol drops for a few more days to help prevent infection and lubricate the eye.

Recurrent abrasions — Occasionally the corneal epithelium may repeatedly break down where there has been a previous injury or there is an inherently weak adhesion between the epithelial cells and the basement membrane. These recurrences usually occur at night when there is little secretion of tears and the epithelium may be torn off. Treatment is long term and entails drops during the day and ointment at night to lubricate the eye. Occasionally, a surgical procedure may be carried out to enhance the adhesion between the epithelium and the underlying basement membrane.

Foreign bodies

It is important to identify and remove conjunctival and corneal foreign bodies. A patient may not recall a foreign body having entered the eye, so it is essential to be on the lookout for a foreign body if a patient has an uncomfortable red eye. It may be necessary to use local anaesthetic both to examine the eye and to remove the foreign body. Although patients often request them, local anaesthetics should never be given to patients to use themselves, because they impede healing, and further injury may occur to an anaesthetised eye.

Small loose conjunctival foreign bodies can be removed with the edge of a tissue or a cotton wool bud, or they can be washed out with water. The upper lid must be everted to exclude a subtarsal foreign body, particularly if there are corneal scratches or a continuing feeling that a foreign body is present. However, this should not be done if a penetrating injury is present. Corneal foreign bodies are often more difficult to remove if they are metallic for they are often "rusted on". They must be removed as they will prevent healing and rust may permanently stain the cornea. A cotton wool bud or the edge of a piece of cardboard can be used. If this does not work, a needle tip (or special rotary drill) can be used, but great care must be taken when using these as the eye may easily be damaged. If there is any doubt, these patients should be referred to an ophthalmologist. When the foreign body has been removed any remaining epithelial defect can be treated as an abrasion.

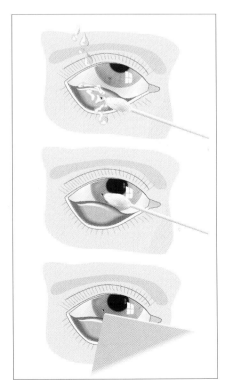

Removal of a foreign body from the eye.

Removal of a foreign body.

- Use local anaesthetic
- If the foreign body is loose, irrigate the eye
- If the foreign body is adherent, use a cotton wool bud or the edge of a piece of cardboard

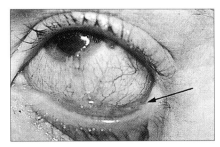

Lower lid gently pulled down to show a conjunctival foreign body. The cornea has also been perforated.

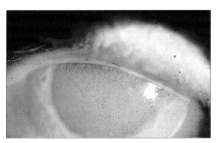

Cornea after welding damage stained with fluorescein and illuminated with blue light.

Dealing with chemical damage to the eye.

- Immediately wash out eye with water
- Remove loose particles
- Refer patient to ophthalmic department
- BEWARE ALKALIS

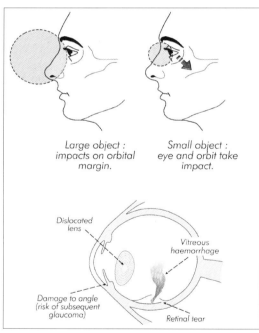

Complications of blunt trauma to the eye.

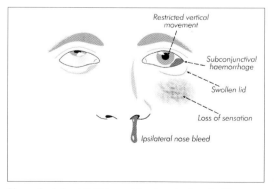

Signs of a left orbital blowout fracture (patient looking upwards).

Radiation damage

The commonest form of radiation damage occurs when welding has been carried out without adequate shielding of the eye. The corneal epithelium is damaged by the ultraviolet rays and the patient typically presents with painful, weeping eyes some hours after welding. Radiation damage can also occur after exposure to large amounts of reflected sunlight; for example, snow blindness. Treatment is as for a corneal abrasion.

Chemical damage

If chemicals are splashed into the eye, the eye and the conjunctival sacs (fornices) should immediately be washed out with copious amounts of water. Alkalis are particularly damaging, and any loose bits such as lime should be removed from the conjunctival sac, with the aid of local anaesthetic if necessary. The patient should then be referred immediately to an ophthalmic department. If there is any doubt irrigation should be continued for as long as possible.

Blunt injuries

If a large object (such as a football) hits the eye most of the impact is usually taken by the orbital margin. If a smaller object (such as a squash ball) hits the area the eye itself may take most of the impact.

Haemorrhage may occur and a collection of blood may be plainly visible in the anterior chamber of the eye (hyphaema). Patients who sustain such injuries need to be reviewed at an eye unit as the pressure in the eye may rise, and further haemorrhages may require surgical intervention. Haemorrhage may also occur into the vitreous or in the retina, and this may be accompanied by a retinal detachment. All patients with visual impairment after blunt injury should be seen in an ophthalmic department.

The pupil may also be damaged and react poorly to light. This is particularly important in a patient with an associated head injury, as this may be interpreted as (or mask) the dilated pupil that is suggestive of an acute extradural haematoma. The lens may be damaged or dislocated and a cataract may develop. Damage to the drainage angle of the eye (which cannot be seen without a mirror contact lens and a slit lamp microscope) increases the chances of glaucoma developing in later life.

If the force of impact is transmitted to the orbit, an orbital fracture may occur (usually in the floor, which is thin and has little support). Clues to the presence of an inferior "blow out" fracture include diplopia, a recessed eye, defective eye movements (especially vertical), an ipsilateral nose bleed, and diminished sensation over the distribution of the infraorbital nerve. The fracture may need repair and these patients should be referred to an ophthalmic department.

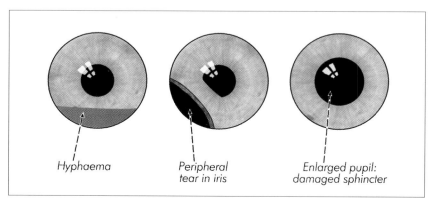

Signs of damage to the eye itself.

Penetrating injuries and eyelid lacerations

Lacerations of the eyelids need specialist attention if:
- *the lid margins have been torn* — these must be sewn together accurately;
- *the lacrimal ducts have been damaged* — the cut ends must be reapposed;
- *there is any suspicion of a foreign body or penetrating eyelid injury* — objects may easily penetrate the orbit, and even the cranial cavity through the orbit.

Penetrating injuries of the eye can easily be missed because they may seal themselves, and the signs of abnormality are subtle. Any history of a high velocity injury (particularly a hammer and chisel injury) should lead one strongly to suspect a penetrating injury. In that case, the eye should be examined very gently and no pressure should be brought to bear on the globe.

Signs to look for include a distorted pupil, cataract, and vitreous haemorrhage. The pupil should be dilated (if there is no head injury) and a thorough search made for an intraocular foreign body. If in doubt, a radiograph of the orbit should be taken.

If the eye is clearly perforated it should be protected from any pressure and the patient sent immediately to the nearest eye department.

Penetrating eye injuries — beware:

- Hammer and chisel
- Glass
- Knives
- Thorns
- Darts
- Pencils

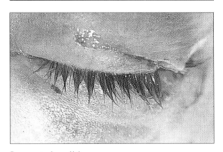

Lacerated eyelid.

5 Acute visual disturbance

Acute disturbance of vision in a non-inflamed eye demands an accurate history, as the patient may have only just noticed a longstanding visual defect. The range of diagnoses and urgency of treatment depend on this assessment. Acute visual disturbance of unknown cause requires urgent referral.

Symptoms and signs

In many cases the diagnosis can be made from the history. Symptoms of floaters or flashing lights suggest a vitreous detachment, a vitreous haemorrhage, or a retinal detachment. Horizontal field loss usually indicates a retinal vascular problem, whereas a vertical defect suggests an abnormality posterior to the optic chiasm. If there is central field loss ("I can't see things in the centre") there may be a disorder at the macula. Associated symptoms such as headache may indicate giant cell arteritis or migraine.

The visual acuity gives a strong clue to the diagnosis. A total lack of perception of light indicates complete occlusion of the central retinal artery or the arteries supplying the head of the optic nerve. The nature of the field defect gives clues as outlined above.

Obstruction of the red reflex on ophthalmoscopy suggests a vitreous haemorrhage, although the patient may have a pre-existing cataract.

The appearance of the macula, remaining retina, and head of the optic nerve will indicate the diagnosis if there has been haemorrhage or arterial or venous occlusion in these areas.

History and examination in the patient with acute visual disturbance.

History

- Floaters
- Field loss
- Zigzag lines
- Flashing lights
- Headache
- Pain on moving eye

Examination

- Acuity
- Pupil reactions
- Appearance of retina, macula, and optic nerve
- Red reflex
- Field loss

Causes and features of acute visual disturbance (in an uninflamed eye).

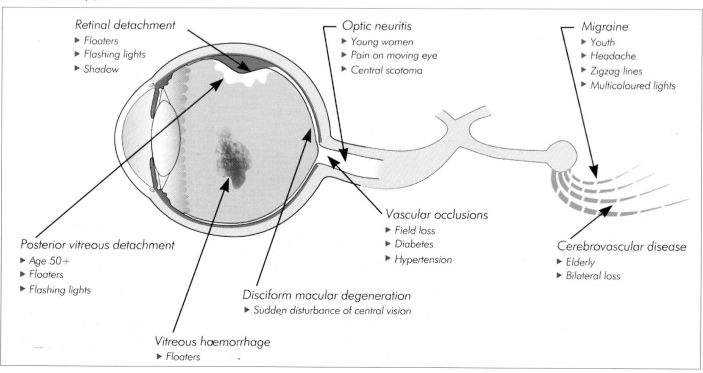

Retinal detachment
- Floaters
- Flashing lights
- Shadow

Optic neuritis
- Young women
- Pain on moving eye
- Central scotoma

Migraine
- Youth
- Headache
- Zigzag lines
- Multicoloured lights

Posterior vitreous detachment
- Age 50+
- Floaters
- Flashing lights

Vascular occlusions
- Field loss
- Diabetes
- Hypertension

Cerebrovascular disease
- Elderly
- Bilateral loss

Disciform macular degeneration
- Sudden disturbance of central vision

Vitreous haemorrhage
- Floaters

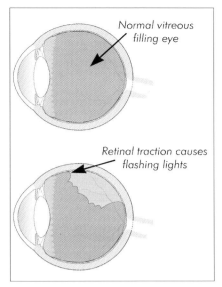

Posterior vitreous detachment causing retinal traction and a "flashing lights" sensation.

Posterior vitreous detachment

Posterior vitreous detachment is the most common cause of acute onset of floaters, particularly with advancing age, and is one of the most common causes of acute visual disturbance.

History — The patient presents complaining of floaters. In posterior vitreous detachment the vitreous body collapses and detaches from the retina. If there are associated flashing lights it suggests that there may be traction on the retina, which may result in a retinal hole and a subsequent retinal detachment.

Examination — The visual acuity is characteristically normal, and there should be no loss of visual field.

Management — If there is any doubt about the precise diagnosis the patient should be referred to an ophthalmologist on the same day so that an associated retinal hole or detachment may be excluded. The patient may require a further visit one to two months later to exclude subsequent development of a retinal hole.

Vitreous haemorrhage

History — The patient complains of a sudden onset of floaters, or "blobs", in the vision. The visual acuity may be normal or, if the haemorrhage is dense, it may be reduced. Flashing lights indicate retinal traction and are a dangerous symptom. Haemorrhage may occur from spontaneous rupture of vessels, avulsion of vessels during retinal traction, or bleeding from abnormal new vessels. If the patient is shortsighted, retinal detachment is more likely. If there is associated diabetes mellitus the patient may have bled from new vessels.

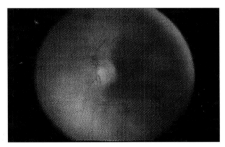

Vitreous haemorrhage.

Examination — The visual acuity depends on the extent of haemorrhage. Projection of light is accurate unless the haemorrhage is extremely severe. Ophthalmoscopy shows the red reflex to be reduced; there may be clots of blood that move with the vitreous.

Management — The patient should be referred to an ophthalmologist to exclude a retinal detachment. Ultrasound examination of the eye may be useful, particularly if the haemorrhage precludes a view of the retina. Underlying causes such as diabetes must also be excluded. If a vitreous haemorrhage fails to clear spontaneously the patient may benefit from having the vitreous removed (vitrectomy).

Retinal detachment

Retinal detachment should be suspected from the history. It is only when the detachment is advanced that the vision and the visual fields are affected and the detachment becomes readily visible on direct ophthalmoscopy.

History — The patient may complain of a sudden onset of floaters, indicating pigment or blood in the vitreous, and flashing lights caused by traction on the retina. These, however, are not invariable and the patient may not present until there is field loss when the area of detachment is sufficiently large, or a deterioration in visual acuity if the macula is detached. Retinal detachment is more likely to occur if the retina is thin (in the shortsighted patient), damaged (by trauma), or the ocular dynamics have been disturbed (by a previous cataract operation). Traction from a contracting membrane after vitreous haemorrhage in patient with diabetes can also cause a retinal detachment.

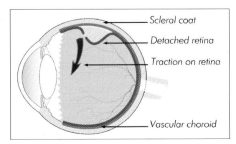

Retinal detachment. Only when advanced is detachment visible on direct ophthalmoscopy.

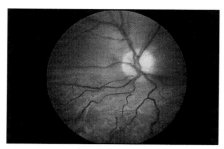

Detached retinal folds — inferior detachment.

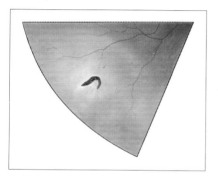

Retinal tear.

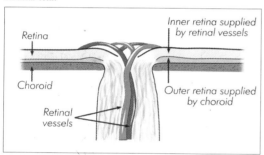

Retina

Choroid

Retinal vessels

Inner retina supplied by retinal vessels

Outer retina supplied by choroid

Blood supply of retina

Arterial occlusion.
Infarction of lower half of retina (below).
Embolus (below, right).
Ischaemic optic nerve head, pale and swollen (below, far right).

Examination — The visual acuity is normal if the macula is still attached, but the acuity is reduced to counting fingers or hand movements if the macula is detached. Field loss (not complete in the early stages) is dependent on the size and location of the detachment. Direct ophthalmoscopy will not detect the abnormality if the detachment is small; detached retinal folds may be seen in larger detachments.

Management — The patient should be referred urgently. Only small retinal holes with no associated fluid under the retina can be treated with a laser, which causes an inflammatory reaction that seals the hole. True detachments usually require an operation to seal any holes, reduce vitreous traction, and if necessary drain fluid from beneath the neuroretina. A vitrectomy may be required, and this is carried out using fine microsurgical cutting instruments inserted into the eye with fibreoptic illumination. This may be combined with the use of special intraocular gases (e.g. sulphur hexafluoride) or silicone oil to keep the retina flat. If gas is used the patient may have to posture face down, and cannot travel by air (the intraocular gas expands at altitude) until most of the gas in the eye has been absorbed, which may take several weeks.

Arterial occlusion

History — The patient complains of a sudden onset of visual disturbance. This may be temporary (amaurosis fugax) if the obstruction dislodges, or permanent. It is often described as a "curtain" descending over the vision.

Examination — The visual acuity depends on whether the macula or its fibres are affected. There may be no direct pupillary reaction if there is a complete occlusion. The extent of field loss depends on the area of retina affected. The retinal artery and its branches supply the inner two thirds of the neuroretina, and the outer third is supplied by the choroid. The arteries may be blocked by atherosclerosis, thrombosis, or emboli, and the attacks may be associated with a history of transient ischaemic attacks if the aetiology is embolic. When the retina infarcts it becomes oedematous and pale and masks the choroidal circulation except at the macula, which is extremely thin — hence the "cherry red spot" appearance. Ophthalmoscopy may be normal initially, before oedema is established. Plaques of cholesterol or calcium may occasionally be seen in the vessels.

Management — Giant cell arteritis must be excluded by the history, examination, and by checking the erythrocyte sedimentation rate. Emboli from the carotid arteries and heart should be excluded. Attempts may be made to open up the arterial circulation in acute cases by ocular massage, or by carbon dioxide rebreathing to cause arterial dilatation. Factors predisposing to vascular disease (for example, smoking, diabetes and hyperlipidaemia) should be identified and treated.

   Occlusion of the posterior ciliary arteries may cause ischaemia and infarction of the head of the optic nerve (ischaemic optic neuropathy). The nerve head swells and this may be mistaken for papilloedema. Papilloedema, however, is usually bilateral and the visual acuity is not affected until late in its development. In addition, the optic disc in ischaemic optic neuropathy is pale because of the lack of blood perfusion. Giant cell arteritis must be excluded in these cases as the other eye may also go blind if intravenous and oral steroid treatment is not started promptly.

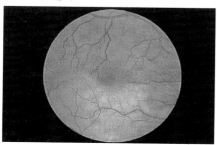

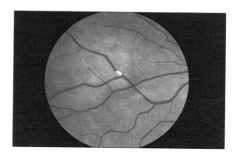

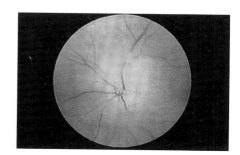

Venous occlusion

History — The visual acuity will be disturbed only if the occlusion affects the temporal arcades and damages the macula. Patients may otherwise complain only of a vague visual disturbance or of field loss. The arteries and veins share a common sheath in the eye, and venous occlusion most commonly occurs where arteries and veins cross, and in the head of the nerve. Thus raised arterial pressure can give rise to venous occlusion. Hyperviscosity (for example, in myeloma) and increased "stickiness" of the blood (as in diabetes mellitus) will also predispose to venous occlusion. This leads to haemorrhages and oedema of the retina. Occlusion of the central retinal vein within the head of the nerve leads to swelling of the optic disc.

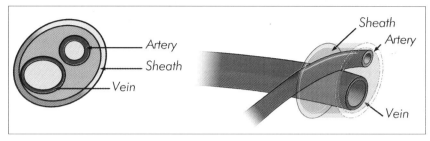

Raised blood pressure causes thickening of arteries leading to compression of veins.

Examination — Visual acuity will not be affected unless the macula is damaged. There may only be some peripheral field loss if a branch occlusion has occurred. Ophthalmoscopy shows characteristic flame haemorrhages in the affected areas, with a swollen disc if there is occlusion of the central vein. An afferent pupillary defect and retinal cotton wool spots imply an ischaemic, damaged retina and are a bad prognostic sign.

Management — Hypertension, diabetes mellitus, hyperviscosity and glaucoma must be identified and treated if present. If the retina becomes ischaemic it stimulates the formation of new vessels on the iris (rubeosis) and subsequent neovascularisation of the angle may lead to secondary glaucoma. Fluorescein angiography may be useful. This involves the injection of intravenous fluorescein and sequential fundus photography with light filters, to identify areas of poor perfusion and fluorescein leakage. Laser treatment is used to ablate the ischaemic retina in an attempt to prevent new vessel formation.

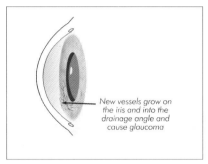

New vessels grow on the iris and into the drainage angle and cause glaucoma

Neovascularisation of the iris induced by vasoproliferative factors released from the ischaemic retina.

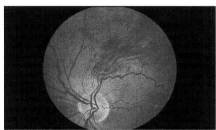

Branch retinal vein occlusion.

Disciform macular degeneration

History — The patient notices a sudden disturbance of central vision. Straight lines may seem wavy and objects may be distorted, even seeming larger or smaller than normal. Eventually, central vision may be completely lost. This central area of visual distortion or loss moves as the patient tries to look around it. The layer under the retina is the black retinal pigment epithelium. Most commonly with increasing age (the patient is normally over 60) and in certain conditions (for example, high myopia) neovascular membranes may develop under this layer in the macular region. These membranes may leak fluid or bleed causing an acute disturbance of vision.

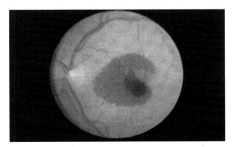

Leakage of fluid at macula (right eye).

Macular haemorrhage (left eye).

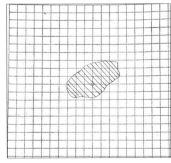

Amsler grid: distortion in patient with age related macular degeneration.

Examination — The visual acuity depends on the extent of macula involvement. If the patient looks at a grid pattern (Amsler chart) the lines may look distorted centrally. The peripheral fields are normal. On fundal examination the macula may look normal, or there may be a raised area within it. Haemorrhage in the retina is red but it appears black if it is under the retinal pigment epithelium. There may be associated deposits of yellow degenerative retinal products (drusen).

Management — Some cases are treatable with a laser that occludes these neovascular membranes, which are identified with fluorescein angiography. If a patient has had a subretinal neovascular membrane in one eye that has destroyed central vision, they are at risk of the same thing occurring in the other eye. The problem with laser treatment is that it may cause immediate worsening of vision with benefit only in the long term. Trials are still underway to determine the role of radiation therapy to prevent the progression of the neovascular membranes.

Retrobulbar neuritis

History — The patient is usually a woman aged 20 to 40 who complains of a disturbance of vision in one eye. There is usually pain that worsens on movement of the eye. The visual acuity may range from 6/6 to perception of light. Despite a "normal" visual acuity, the patient usually has an afferent pupillary defect and may notice that the colour red looks faded when viewed with the affected eye (red desaturation). The field defect is usually a central field loss (central scotoma). It is extremely important to test the field of the other eye as a field defect may suggest a lesion further back (for example, a pituitary adenoma). The optic disc is swollen if the "inflammation" is anterior in the nerve. There may have been previous attacks. Accompanying symptoms of general demyelinating disease (such as pins and needles, weakness, incontinence) suggest multiple sclerosis.

Management — Most patients recover spontaneously, but they may be left with diminished acuity and optic atrophy. Treatment with systemic steroids does not alter the long term visual prognosis but may hasten recovery. Systemic steroids may, in selected patients, reduce the incidence of subsequent multiple sclerosis. Referral to a neurologist is necessary. If there is doubt about the diagnosis, the patient may need further investigation to exclude a space occupying lesion.

Cardiovascular disease

History — The patient may have a hemiparesis on the same side as the visual field loss. Patients sometimes complain of "the beginning or end of a line of print disappearing", and some may complain of a decrease in acuity. The visual pathways pass through a large area of the cerebral hemispheres, and any vascular occlusion in these areas will affect these pathways. Lesions behind the chiasm are the most common and lead to contralateral field loss in both eyes which respects the vertical. This is in contrast to vascular lesions in the eye or optic nerve which either affect the whole field of one eye, or if partial tend to respect the horizontal meridian in that eye. More posteriorly placed lesions in the brain tend to spare the macula vision in the affected fields.

Examination — The visual acuity should be preserved, though patients may say half the Snellen chart is missing, in which case the appropriate bilateral visual field loss is present.

Treatment — It is important to make the diagnosis and exclude any underlying cause for vascular disease such as diabetes or hypertension. The field defects sometimes improve with time, and patients should be taught to compensate for their field defect with appropriate head and eye movements.

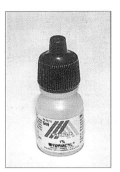
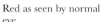
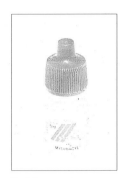

Red as seen by normal eye.

Red desaturation.

> **Treatment with steroids does not alter the visual prognosis, but may hasten recovery in retrobulbar neuritis**

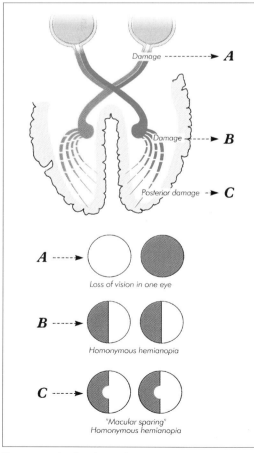

Loss of vision in one eye

Homonymous hemianopia

"Macular sparing" Homonymous hemianopia

Damage to visual pathways from vascular lesions.

Migraine

History — Migraine may initially present with symptoms of visual loss. The features are well known and include:

- *a family history of migraine*;
- *attacks set off by certain stimuli* — for example, particular foods;
- *fortification spectra in both eyes* — these include zig zag lines and multicoloured flashes of light;
- *associated headache and nausea* — though these symptoms may not be present).

Examination — The patient may have a bilateral field defect but this usually resolves within a few hours.

Management — Conventional treatment with analgesics and antiemetics may be necessary. Long term prophylaxis may be required if attacks occur frequently.

Migraine — particular visual features.

- Zigzag lines
- Multicoloured flashing lights

6 Cataracts

Cataracts may cause difficulty in:

- Reading
- Recognising faces
- Watching television
- Seeing in bright light
- Driving

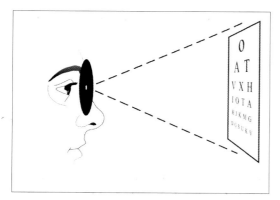

A pinhole improves the visual acuity if the problem is caused by refractive error.

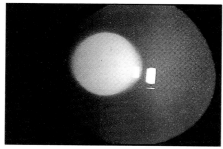

Clear red reflex.

"Cataract" is the term used to describe any lens opacity from the smallest dot to complete opacification. The prevalence of cataracts increases with age; 65% of people aged 50 to 59 have opacities and all of those aged over 80. Only when the opacities significantly interfere with vision is an operation contemplated. Cataracts are the most important cause of blindness in the world today.

Symptoms

Symptoms depend on whether the cataracts are unilateral or bilateral and the degree and position of the opacity. If the cataract is unilateral the patient may not notice its effects until he has cause to cover the good eye. Patients may complain of difficulty in reading (which should be differentiated from presbyopia that is normal with older people), in recognising faces, and watching television. They may complain that their vision worsens in bright light, especially if their opacity is central. Occasionally patients experience monocular diplopia and see haloes around lights; this occurs because the lens opacity interferes with light rays passing to the back of the eye. Some patients may even report that they can read without glasses. This happens when a nuclear sclerotic cataract increases the converging power of the lens, so making the patient myopic (shortsighted).

Signs

The signs of cataract are as follows:

A reduction in visual acuity — The degree of visual impairment depends on the nature of the cataract and the conditions of testing. Visual acuity should also be tested with a pin hole to eliminate the effect of refractive errors.

A diminished red reflex on ophthalmoscopy — When the ophthalmoscope is used to view the eye from about two feet away, the reflection of the fundus can be seen as a "red reflex". This is the troublesome reflex so often seen in photographs of people taken with a flashlight. If there is any opacity between the cornea and the retina this reflex will have opacities in it. The nature of the opacities in the reflex will depend on the position and extent of the opacities in the optical media. This reflex is more easily seen when the pupil is dilated.

A change in the appearance of the lens — If one shines a bright light on the eye the lens may appear brown, or even white if the cataract is more advanced.

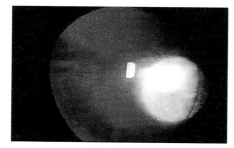

Opacities obscuring red reflex.

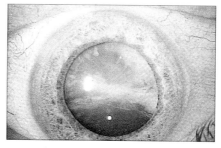

Cortical cataract.

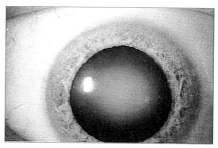

Nuclear sclerotic cataract.

Although cataracts are common, they are not the only cause of visual problems. The patient with a cataract should be able to point to the position of a light. Lack of normal "projection of light" should lead one to suspect problems either in the posterior part of the eye or beyond. The pupillary reactions should also be normal. If they are not, retinal disease or an abnormality of the visual pathway should be suspected.

Cataracts occurring in children are much more serious, as the development of the vision may be irreversibly impaired (visual deprivation amblyopia) even if the cataracts are removed later. Any child with suspected cataracts should be referred immediately. Cataracts in young children are detected by looking at the red reflex, and this should be a routine part of the examination of a young child.

Children with cataracts must be referred immediately

Causes

There are many conditions that are associated with cataracts. Changes within the lens associated with ageing are, however, the most common cause of cataract. Cataracts also occur more often in patients with diabetes, uveitis and a history of trauma to the eye. Prolonged courses of steroids, both oral and topical, can also give rise to cataracts. Children with cataracts need to be investigated to exclude treatable metabolic conditions such as galactosaemia.

Causes of cataract include:

- Age
- Diabetes
- Inflammation
- Trauma
- Steroids

Management

There is no effective medical treatment for established cataracts. The treatment is surgical.

Indications for operation
The decision to operate depends primarily on the effect of the cataracts on the patient's vision. With advances in operative technique, surgery can be carried out at any stage with minimal risk. There is no set level below which an operation is essential, but most patients with a vision of 6/18 or worse in both eyes because of lens opacities benefit from cataract extraction. Some elderly patients, however, may be perfectly happy with this level of vision. Simple advice such as the recommendation to use a good reading light that provides illumination from above and behind, may be adequate.

On the other hand, a younger patient with more exacting visual demands may opt for an operation much earlier. (The minimum standard for driving is about 6/10; this is equivalent to a line between 6/9 and 6/12.) With certain types of cataract, such as an opacity located at the back of the lens (posterior subcapsular cataract) the vision may be 6/6 in dim conditions when the pupil is dilated. However, in bright sunlight the pupil constricts and most of the light entering the eye has to pass through this opacity causing glare and a fall in acuity. Surgery would be performed if the patient was disabled by this even though the tested vision was 6/6. On the whole, the surgeon's advice is tailored to the individual patient. Many years ago surgeons waited until the cataract was mature or "ripe" (when the contents became liquified) because this made aspiration of the contents of the lens easier. With advances in microsurgery, however, there is now no longer any need to wait for the cataract to mature.

Cataract surgery with lens implantations can be combined with other intraocular surgery if necessary including glaucoma drainage or corneal graft surgery.

Technique of operation
"Phacoemulsification" method — Most cataract surgery in the United Kingdom is now performed using this method. A very small tunnel incision (approximately 3 mm) is made in the eye and a circular hole (diameter approximately 5 mm) is made in the anterior capsule of the lens (capsulorhexis). A fine ultrasonic probe is then used to liquefy the hard lens nucleus (phaecoemulsification) through this hole. Any remaining soft lens

Cataract surgery

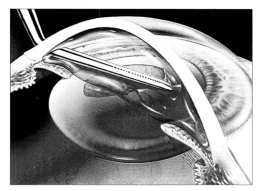

Removal of the anterior capsule of the lens.

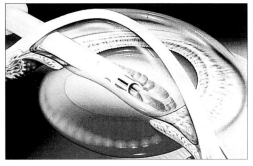

Liquefaction of lens nucleus with an ultrasonic probe through a 3 mm incision.

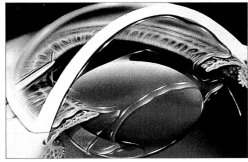

Plastic lens being inserted into the remaining clear capsular bag of the natural lens.

Intracapsular cataract surgery

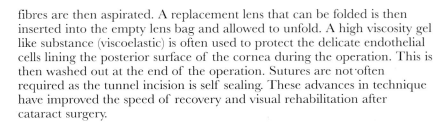

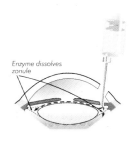

Enzyme dissolves
zonule

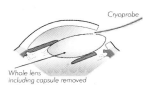

Cryoprobe

Whole lens
including capsule removed

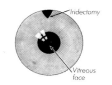

Iridectomy

Vitreous
face

fibres are then aspirated. A replacement lens that can be folded is then inserted into the empty lens bag and allowed to unfold. A high viscosity gel like substance (viscoelastic) is often used to protect the delicate endothelial cells lining the posterior surface of the cornea during the operation. This is then washed out at the end of the operation. Sutures are not often required as the tunnel incision is self sealing. These advances in technique have improved the speed of recovery and visual rehabilitation after cataract surgery.

Extracapsular method — This was, until recently, the most popular method of cataract extraction. An incision is made in the eye, and the anterior capsule is cut open with the tip of a sharp needle. The large nucleus is then expressed whole and the remaining soft lens fibres aspirated. A non-folding lens is then inserted into the empty lens bag and the incision closed with fine sutures.

Intracapsular method — In this method, the entire lens is removed within its capsule, usually with a cryoprobe, after the suspensory ligaments of the lens have been dissolved by the enzyme chymotrypsin. As there is no remnant lens capsule the vitreous gel in the eye can move forward and block the flow of aqueous through the pupil. A hole cut in the iris (iridectomy) allows the aqueous to bypass the pupil. This method is now usually used only in special situations.

Anaesthesia

For most patients, cataract surgery is now carried out under local anaesthesia as a day case. Local anaesthetic can be injected around the eye, but with modern closed-system, small-incision cataract surgery, the operation can be carried out safely in selected patients with just topical (eyedrops) anaesthesia. Occasionally, intraocular (intracameral) local anaesthesia is used.

Intraocular lens implants

The final refractive state of the eye after operation can be chosen by measuring the curvature of the cornea (keratometry) and the length of the eye (ultrasound biometry), and then implanting a lens of appropriate power. An intraocular lens implant has the optical advantage of being placed in the eye in the position of its natural counterpart, thus overcoming the optical problems associated with spectacles and contact lenses. Myopia and hypermetropia can be corrected during cataract surgery by inserting an appropriately powered intraocular lens. However, patients still usually require glasses for reading or distance as implanted lenses have a fixed focus.

Most lenses implanted nowadays are posterior chamber lenses, which are placed in the empty lens bag, after the lens contents have been removed from the eye. With this type of lens the lens implant sits in a natural position. These lenses can be folded and inserted through a minute incision (2–3 mm). If the lens capsule is not present or cannot support a posterior chamber lens unaided, the lens can be sutured in place. Alternatively, an anterior chamber lens, which is supported in the anterior chamber angle, can be used. In the past, iris clip lenses were used although they are not used now. The pupil should not be dilated if the iris clip type of lens has been used as the lens may dislocate.

Feet of implant
rest in angle

Implant clips onto
pupil margin

Lens sits in
capsular bag

Anterior chamber
implant

Iris clip lens

Posterior chamber
implant

Rarely used

Different types of lens implants.

Postoperative care after cataract surgery.

- Steroid drops (inflammation)
- Antibiotic drops (infection)
- Avoid very strenuous exertion and ocular trauma

Postoperative care

Most patients are treated for several weeks with steroid drops to reduce inflammation and antibiotic drops to prevent infection. Patients have traditionally been advised to avoid activities that may significantly raise the pressure in the eyeball such as strenuous exercise or heavy lifting for a few weeks after the operation. However, with modern small incision surgery patients are returning to normal activities within a few days of surgery. If sutures have been necessary, then these often have to be taken out before spectacles can be prescribed because of the changes they induce in the shape and refractive state of the eye.

The remaining lens capsule may thicken (usually over months or years) and this may need to be cut open. In patients who have had previous cataract surgery, capsular thickening is the commonest cause of gradually worsening vision. Division of this thickened capsule (capsulotomy) is usually done with a special laser (called the Q-switched Neodymium Yttrium-Aluminium-Garnett or Nd-YAG laser) that creates microscopic focused explosions that dissect tissue rather than burning it. This avoids the need to open the eye surgically, and can be performed painlessly (the capsule has no pain fibres) on an outpatient basis, under topical anaesthesia, with the patient sitting at a slit-lamp microscope. This has given rise to the commonly held misconception by patients that cataracts can be removed by laser alone.

Optical correction after operation

Removal of the crystalline lens results in an eye with a large hypermetropic refractive error. This refractive error is now usually corrected with an intraocular lens implant at the time of surgery. If an implant has been inserted resulting in clear vision for distance, glasses will usually still be required for reading fine print, as the new lens has a fixed focus. Intraocular lenses that allow several points of focus (multifocal intraocular lenses) are available, but possible problems include a suboptimal visual acuity and a reduction in perception of contrast. Therefore, single focus intraocular lenses are normally used. However, if this is not possible for technical reasons, or the patient has had a cataract extraction done before intraocular lenses were commonly used, optical correction has to be achieved with spectacles or a contact lens.

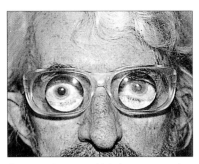

Cataract glasses — thick, heavy, expensive, with magnified image and reduced field of vision — are now rarely necessary because of intraocular lens implants.

Spectacles — The natural lens has great refractive power and consequently the spectacles required to correct the refractive error after cataract extraction are thick and heavy even when they are made of plastic. The corrected image is about 30% larger than that seen by the normal eye. This means that the image from an eye that has had a cataract removed with subsequent spectacle correction cannot be fused with the other eye, unless the cataract in the other eye is also removed. Objects are also perceived to be closer than they are, often resulting in accidents — for example, pouring tea into one's lap rather than into the cup. The field of vision is restricted, and there is a "blind" area all round within this field because of the optical aberrations inherent in such powerful lenses. These optical problems do not occur with contact lenses or an intraocular lens implant.

Contact lenses — The size of an image with a contact lens is only 10% larger than the image in the normal eye. The brain can fuse this disparity and thus both an operated eye and an unoperated eye may be used simultaneously. Most patients, however, are elderly and problems may arise in using the contact lens because of an inadequate tear film, difficulties with handling, and infection.

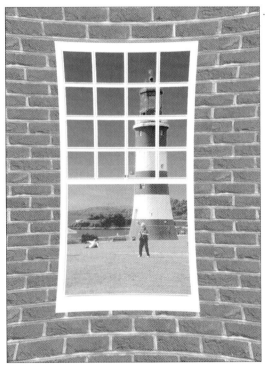

Peripheral image distortion that may be present with cataract spectacles.

Secondary intraocular lens implantation — If the problems posed by using spectacles or contact lenses prove too much, secondary implantation of an intraocular lens can be considered. However, this is not a procedure without risk, particularly in eyes having undergone intracapsular cataract extraction. Complications may occur, including secondary glaucoma. The potential advantages and disadvantages of the various options need to be fully considered by the patient and his ophthalmologist before a final decision is made.

7   Refractive errors

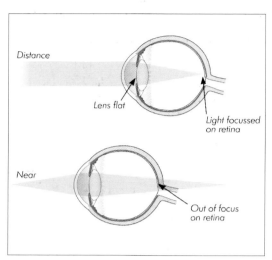

The eye with no refractive error.
Light rays from distant objects are focused on to the retina without the need for accommodation.
Light rays from a close object (e.g. a book) are focused behind the retina. The eye has to accommodate to focus these rays.

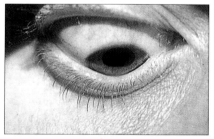

Conical cornea (keratoconus) indenting lower lid on down gaze.

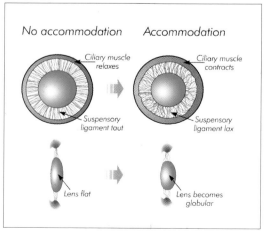

Accommodation: adjustment of the lens of the eye for viewing objects at various distances.

Indistinct vision is most commonly caused by errors of refraction. Doctors do not often have to deal with this problem because patients are usually prescribed glasses by an optometrist. It is extremely important, however, to ask the question: "Is this patient's poor vision caused by a refractive error?

The use of a simple "pinhole" made in a piece of card will help to determine whether or not there is a refractive error. In the absence of disease the vision will improve when the pinhole is used unless the error is extremely large.

The eye with no refractive error

In an eye with no refractive error (emmetropia) light rays from infinity are brought to a focus on the retina by the cornea and lens when the eye is in a "relaxed" state. The cornea contributes about two thirds and the lens one third to the eye's refractive power. Disease affecting the cornea (for example, keratoconus) may cause severe refractive problems.

The rays of light from closer objects such as the printed page are divergent, and have to be brought to a focus on the retina by the process of accommodation. The circular ciliary muscle contracts, allowing the naturally elastic lens to assume a more globular shape that has a greater converging power. In young people the lens is very elastic, but with age the lens gradually hardens and even when the ciliary muscle contracts the lens no longer becomes globular. Thus from the age of 40 onwards close work becomes gradually more difficult (presbyopia). Objects may be held further away to reduce the need for accommodation leading to the complaint "my arms don't seem to be long enough'. Fine detail cannot be discerned.

Convex lenses in the form of reading glasses are therefore needed to converge the light rays from close objects on to the retina. All emmetropic people need reading glasses for close work in later life. People who wear spectacles to see clearly in the distance may find it convenient to change to bifocal lenses in their spectacles when they become presbyopic. In bifocal lenses the reading lens is simply incorporated into the lower part of the spectacle lens. Therefore, the spectacles need not be changed when the individual wants to read. However, details at an intermediate distance such as the prices of items on supermarket shelves are not clear. A third lens segment can be incorporated between that for distance above and that for reading below, creating a trifocal lens. However, many people cannot cope with the "jump" in magnification inherent in the use of these lenses. This has led to the introduction of multifocal lenses in which the lens power increases progressively from top to bottom. People may also have problems adapting to this type of lens as peripheral vision may be distorted.

Eyes do not get worse if a person reads in bad light or does not wear his glasses. The exceptions are young children, who may need a refractive error corrected to prevent amblyopia.

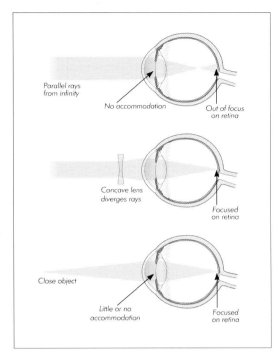

The myopic or shortsighted eye.
Light rays from distant objects are focused in front of the retina, and the lens cannot compensate for this. A concave lens has to be placed in front of the eye to focus the rays on the retina.
Light rays from close objects are focused on the retina with little or no accommodation. Thus, even with loss of accommodation, the myopic eye can read without glasses.

The myopic or shortsighted eye

In the myopic eye light rays from infinity are brought to a focus in front of the retina either because the eye is too long or the converging power of the cornea and lens is too great. To achieve clear vision the rays of light must be diverged by a concave lens so that light rays are focused on the retina.

For near vision, light rays are focused on the retina with little or no accommodation depending on the degree of myopia and the distance at which the object is held. This is the reason that shortsighted people can often read without glasses even late in life, when those without refractive errors need reading glasses.

A certain type of cataract (nuclear sclerosis) increases the refractive power of the lens, making the eye more myopic. Patients with these cataracts may say their reading vision has improved. Patients with an extreme degree of short-sightedness are more susceptible to retinal detachment, macular degeneration, and primary open angle glaucoma.

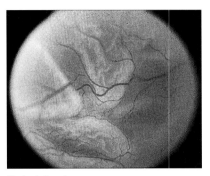

Retinal detachment.

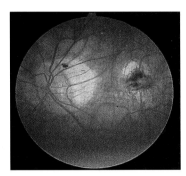

Macular degeneration with myopic crescent temporal to disc.

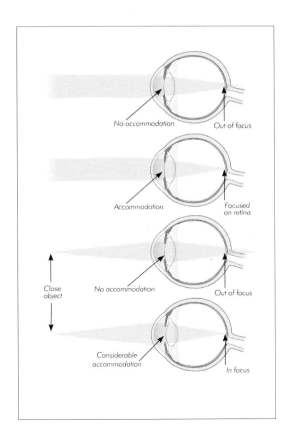

The hypermetropic or longsighted eye.
Light rays from close objects are focused behind the retina. The considerable accommodation required is possible in a young person, but reading glasses are needed in later life.

The hypermetropic or longsighted eye

In the hypermetropic eye, light rays from infinity are brought to a focus behind the retina, either because the eye is too short or because the converging power of the cornea and lens is too weak. Unlike the young shortsighted person, the young longsighted person can achieve a clear retinal image by accommodating. Extremely good distance vision can often be achieved by this "fine tuning" — for example, 6/4 on the Snellen chart — and this has given rise to the term "longsighted". For near vision the longsighted person has to accommodate even more. This may be possible during the first two to three decades of life, but the need for reading glasses arises earlier than in the normal person. Typically, the longsighted person needs reading glasses at about 30 years of age. If a high degree of hypermetropia is present, accommodation may not be adequate, and glasses may have to be worn for both distant and near vision from an earlier age.

As the ability to accommodate (and thus compensate for the hypermetropia) fails with advancing years, the longsighted person may require glasses for both distant and near vision when none were needed before. This may result in the complaint of a deterioration in eyesight because the patient has gone from not needing glasses to needing them for both distance and near vision.

Longsighted people are more susceptible to closed angle glaucoma because their smaller eyes are more likely to have shallow anterior chambers and narrow angles.

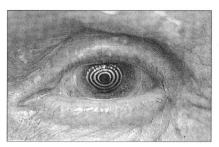

Reflections of concentric circles showing distortion by astigmatic cornea.

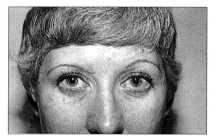

Gas permeable contact lenses to correct myopia.

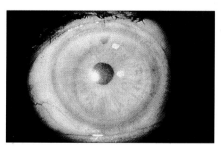

Soft contact lens fitted after cataract extraction.

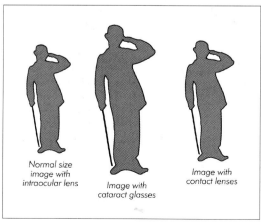

Normal size image with intraocular lens

Image with cataract glasses

Image with contact lenses

Different sized images with different types of optical correction after cataract surgery.

The astigmatic eye

Astigmatism occurs when the cornea does not have an even curvature. A good analogy is that of a soccer ball (no astigmatism) and a rugby ball (astigmatism). The curvature of a normal cornea may be likened to that of the back of a ladle and that of the astigmatic eye to the back of a spoon. This uneven curvature results in an uneven focus in different meridians, and the eye cannot compensate by accommodating.

Astigmatism can be corrected by a lens that has power in only one meridian (a cylinder). Alternatively, an evenly curved surface may be achieved by fitting a hard contact lens. Astigmatism can be caused by any disease that affects the shape of the cornea; for example, a meibomian cyst may press hard enough on the cornea to cause distortion.

Contact lenses

Contact lenses have become increasingly popular in recent years. There are several types, which can be grouped into three categories.

Hard lenses are made of polymethylmethacrylate (plastic material) and not permeable to gases or liquids. They cannot be worn continuously because the cornea becomes hypoxic and they are the most difficult lenses to get used to. Because of their rigidity, however, they correct astigmatism well and are durable. Infection and allergy are less likely with this type of lens. They are now less commonly prescribed, but there are still many people who have been using this type of lens for a long time with no problems.

Gas permeable lenses have properties between those of hard and soft lenses. They allow the passage of oxygen through to the tear film and the cornea, and they are better tolerated than hard lenses. Being semi-rigid they correct astigmatism better than soft lenses. They are, however, more prone to the accumulation of deposits and are also less durable than hard lenses. Gas permeable lenses are usually used as daily wear lenses.

Soft lenses have a high water content and are permeable to both gases and liquids. They are tolerated much better than hard or gas permeable lenses and they can be worn for much longer periods. Both infection and allergy, however, are more common. The lenses are also less durable, are more prone to the accumulation of deposits, and do not correct astigmatism as well as do the harder lenses. Nevertheless, because they are so well tolerated they are now the most commonly prescribed lenses.

Certain types of gas permeable and soft lenses can be worn continuously for up to several months because of their high oxygen permeability, but the risk of sight threatening complications is higher than with daily wear lenses.

Disposable lenses are soft lenses that are designed to be thrown away after a short period of continuous use. They are popular because no cleaning is required during this period. However, it is important that the lenses are used as recommended, or the risk of complications such corneal infection rise significantly.

Indications for prescribing contact lenses

Personal appearance and the inconvenience of spectacles are common reasons for prescribing contact lenses. They may also considerably reduce the optical aberrations that are associated with the wearing of glasses, particularly those with high power such as are sometimes prescribed for patients who have undergone cataract extraction. The brain cannot resolve the large difference in the size of the retinal images that occurs when the refractive power of the two eyes differs considerably. A good example of this is if a cataract has been removed from only one eye and a spectacle lens has been prescribed, whilst the other eye is normal. A contact lens brings the image size closer to "normal", permitting the brain to fuse the two images. If a person is very myopic, the use of contact lenses rather than spectacles may increase the image size on the retina and improve the visual acuity.

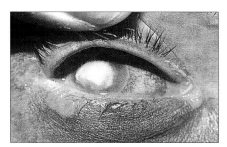

Corneal abscess associated with contact lens wear.

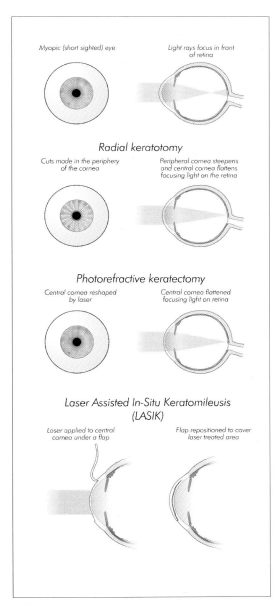

Different types of refractive surgery to correct myopia.

A contact lens also permits irregularities in the cornea to be neutralised, and the effects of an irregularly shaped cornea (for example, keratoconus or following corneal graft surgery) may be corrected.

Relative contraindications to contact lens wear

Contraindications include a history of atopy, "dry eyes", previous glaucoma filtration surgery, and an inability to handle or cope with the management of lenses. These are, however, relative contraindications; a trial of lenses may be the only way to determine whether it is feasible for a particular patient to wear contact lenses.

Complications of wearing contact lenses

The most serious complication of contact lens wear is a corneal abscess. This is most common in elderly patients who have worn soft contact lenses for an extended period. Corneal abrasions are also fairly common.

Any contact lenses wearer with a red eye should have the contact lens removed and the eye stained with fluorescein to show up any corneal abrasion or abscess. **As fluorescein stains soft contact lenses, the eye should be washed out with saline before the lens is replaced. If** there is an abrasion or infection the appropriate treatment should be given, and the contact lens *should not be worn again* until the condition has resolved. The wearing time may have to be built up again, particularly if hard or gas permeable lenses are worn.

Good hygiene is essential for contact lens wearers, to minimise the risks of infection. Lenses should never be licked and replaced in the eye. Non-sterile solutions may contain contaminants such as amoebae, which can lead to intractable ocular infection.

Refractive surgery

There has been much interest in operations to alter the refractive state of the eye, particularly operations to treat myopia. The technique called radial ketatotomy entails making deep radial incisions in the peripheral cornea, which results in flattening of the central cornea and refocusing of light rays nearer the retina. It is only of use in short sight, and possible disadvantages include weakening of the cornea (particularly if the eye subsequently sustains trauma), infection, glare, and fluctuation of the refractive state of the eye. If contact lenses are still required after radial ketatotomy has been performed, they are much more difficult to fit.

A special (excimer) laser has been used to reprofile the surface of the cornea. This laser works by vaporising a very thin layer of the cornea (photoablation), which reshapes the front surface of the cornea, changing its focusing power. This technique is theoretically safer than radial keratotomy, as it does not involve deep cuts into the eye. Side effects include: pain for a few days after the laser treatment; a period when the eye is overcorrected and becomes longsighted; opacification caused by scarring of the treated zone that may result in a reduction of best corrected visual acuity (usually transient); and glare. Predictability of the final refractive result is poor if the patient is very shortsighted. (This is particularly the case if the patient has more than 6 dioptres of myopia).

More recently, a technique called laser-assisted in situ keratomileusis (LASIK) has been introduced. This entails cutting a superficial flap in the cornea, carrying out excimer laser reshaping of the underlying corneal stroma, and then replacing the flap. Advantages of the technique over surface laser treatment include more rapid stabilisation of vision and much better correction of higher degrees of myopia. Disadvantages include complications associated with having to leave a thin delicate layer of cornea to become re-established.

Other laser techniques can also be used to correct astigmatism and hypermetropia, although these are much less commonly used.

If patients are contemplating any type of refractive surgery it is important that they are fully informed of the risks by the operating surgeon, and have time to evaluate the advantages and disadvantages before undergoing a procedure that may cause irreversible change.

8 The glaucomas

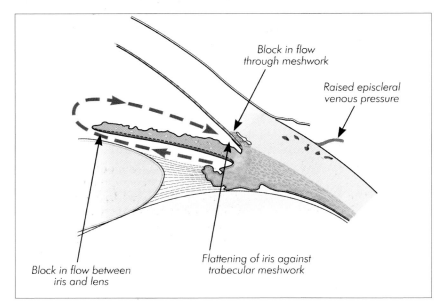

Normal aqueous drainage and possible sites of obstruction.

Block in flow through meshwork

Raised episcleral venous pressure

Block in flow between iris and lens

Flattening of iris against trabecular meshwork

The glaucomas are a range of disorders that are characterised by optic disc cupping, visual field loss, and an intraocular pressure sufficiently raised to damage the eye. This group of disorders is the third most common cause of blindness worldwide.

Normally the ciliary body secretes aqueous, which then flows into the posterior chamber and through the pupil into the anterior chamber. It then leaves the eye through the trabecular meshwork, flowing into the canal of Schlemm and into episcleral veins. The flow and drainage can be obstructed in several ways, as shown in the diagram.

> **The clinical signs of raised intraocular pressure depend on both the rate and degree of the rise in pressure**

Symptoms and signs

The patient with primary open angle glaucoma (also known as chronic open angle glaucoma) may not notice any symptoms until severe visual damage has occurred. This is because the rise in pressure and consequent damage occurs so slowly that the patient has time to compensate. In contrast, the clinical presentation of acute angle closure glaucoma is well known, as the intraocular pressure rises rapidly and results in a red, painful eye with disturbance of vision.

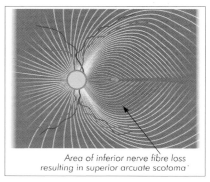

Cloudy cornea after sudden rise in intraocular pressure (acute angle closure glaucoma).

Haloes around lights and a cloudy cornea — The cornea is kept transparent by the continuous removal of fluid by the endothelial cells. If the pressure rises slowly this process takes longer to fail. When the pressure rises quickly (acute closed angle glaucoma) the cornea becomes waterlogged, causing a fall in visual acuity and gives rise to the symptom of haloes (like looking at a light through frosted glass).

Pain — If the rise in pressure is slow, pain is not a feature of glaucoma until the pressure is extremely high. Pain is not characteristically a feature of primary open angle glaucoma.

Field loss — The normal distribution of the retinal nerve fibres is shown in the adjacent diagram. Pressure on the nerve fibres and chronic ischaemia at the head of the nerve cause damage to these fibres and usually result in characteristic patterns of field loss (arcuate scotoma). This, however, spares central vision initially, and the patient does not notice the defect. Sophisticated visual field testing techniques are required to detect early visual field defects. The terminal stage of glaucomatous field loss is a severely contracted field with only a few remaining fibres from the more richly innervated macula area surviving. Even at this stage (tunnel vision) the vision may still be 6/6.

Disc changes — The optic disc marks the exit point of the retinal nerve fibres from the eye. With a sustained rise in pressure the nerve fibres atrophy, leaving the characteristic signs of chronic glaucoma.

Area of inferior nerve fibre loss resulting in superior arcuate scotoma

Normal distribution of nerve fibres in the retina.

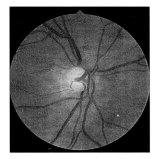

Glaucomatous cupping of optic disc.

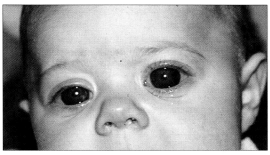

Enlarged watering eyes with cloudy corneas in a child with glaucoma.

Venous occlusion — Raised intraocular pressure can impede blood flow in the low-pressure venous system, predisposing to venous occlusion.

Enlargement of the eye — In the adult no significant enlargement of the eye is possible because growth has ceased. In a young child, however, the eye may expand causing enlargement of the eye (buphthalmos or "ox-eye"). These children may also be photophobic, have watering eyes and cloudy corneas.

Risk factors for glaucomatous damage.

- Level of intraocular pressure
- Increasing age
- Afro-Caribbean origin
- Family history

Primary open angle glaucoma

Primary open angle glaucoma is the most common form of glaucoma and is the third most common cause of registration as blind in the United Kingdom. The resistance to outflow through the trabecular meshwork gradually increases for reasons that are not fully understood, and the pressure in the eye slowly increases causing damage to the nerve. The level of intraocular pressure is the major risk factor for visual loss. There may also be other mechanisms of damage, particularly ischaemia of the optic nerve head.

Symptoms — Because the visual loss is gradual patients do not usually present until severe damage has occurred. The disease can be detected by screening high-risk groups for the signs of glaucoma. At present most patients with primary open angle glaucoma are detected by optometrists at routine examinations.

Groups at risk — The prevalence increases with age from 0.02% in the 40–49 age group to up to 10% in those aged over 80. Those with an increased risk include first degree relatives of patients (one in 10) and people of Afro-Caribbean origin.

Signs — The eye is white and quiet. Field loss is difficult to pick up clinically without specialised equipment until considerable damage (loss of up to 50% of the nerve fibres) has occurred. Computerised field testing equipment may detect nerve fibre damage earlier, particularly if certain types of stimuli such as fine motion or blue on yellow targets are used.

Optic disc changes in glaucoma (left eye).

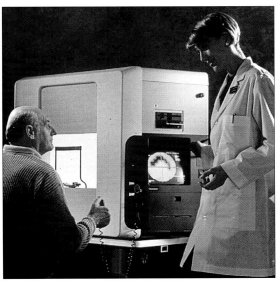

Visual field testing.

Computer assisted field testing is also the best modality for detecting long term change and deterioration of visual fields.

The best signs for the purpose of detection are the disc changes. The cup to disc ratio increases as the nerve fibres atrophy. Asymmetry of disc cupping is also important, as the disease is often more advanced in one eye than the other. Haemorrhages on the optic disc are a poor prognostic sign. Longer term changes in disc cupping are best detected by serial photography, and the more recently introduced scanning laser ophthalmoscope may have greater sensitivity.

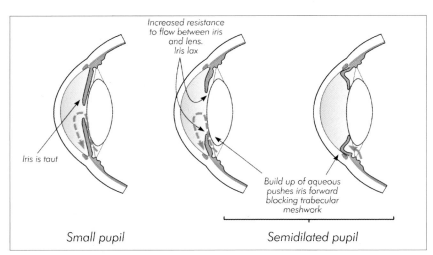

Acute angle closure glaucoma.

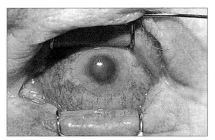

Acute angle closure glaucoma.

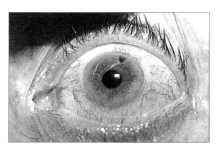

Surgical peripheral iridectomy.

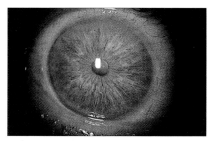

Laser iridotomies.

Acute angle closure glaucoma

Acute angle closure glaucoma is probably the best known type of glaucoma as the presentation is acute and the affected eye becomes red and painful. In angle closure glaucoma apposition of the lens to the back of the iris prevents the flow of aqueous from the posterior chamber to the anterior chamber. This is more likely to occur when the pupil is semi-dilated at night. Aqueous then collects behind the iris and pushes it onto the trabecular meshwork, preventing the drainage of aqueous from the eye, and the intraocular pressure rises rapidly.

Symptoms — The eye becomes red and painful because of the rapid rise in intraocular pressure, and this is often associated with vomiting. Vision is blurred because the cornea is becoming oedematous, and patients may notice haloes around lights because of the dispersion of light. They may give a history of similar attacks in the past that were aborted by going to sleep. During sleep the pupil constricts and may pull the peripheral iris out of the angle.

Groups at risk — This type of glaucoma usually occurs in longsighted people, whose anterior chambers are shallow, and in the elderly, in whom the lens is larger. Women have shallower anterior chambers and are more at risk of this type of glaucoma.

Signs — The visual acuity is impaired, depending on the degree of corneal oedema. The eye is red and tender to touch. The cornea is hazy because of oedema, and the pupil is semi-dilated and fixed to light. The attack begins with the pupil in the semi-dilated position and the rise in pressure makes the iris ischaemic and fixed in that position. On gentle palpation the affected eye feels much harder than the other.

If the patient is seen shortly after an attack has resolved none of these signs may be present, hence the importance of the history.

Management — Emergency treatment is required if the sight of the eye is to be preserved. If it is not possible to get the patient to hospital immediately, actazolamide (Diamox) 500 mg should be given intravenously, and pilocarpine 4% instilled in the eye to constrict the pupil.

The intraocular pressure must first be brought down medically, and a hole must subsequently be made in the peripheral iris, either with a laser or surgically, in order to restore aqueous flow. The other eye should be similarly treated as a prophylactic measure.

If the treatment is delayed adhesions may form between the iris and the cornea (peripheral anterior synechiae) and the trabecular meshwork itself may be damaged. A surgical drainage procedure may then be required.

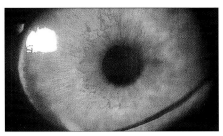

New vessels on the iris causing rubeotic glaucoma.

- **Topical steroids may cause a change in the drainage meshwork resulting in a slow rise in intraocular pressure**
- **Patients may not complain of visual symptoms until severe damage has occurred**

Other types of glaucoma

If there is inflammation in the eye (anterior uveitis) adhesions may develop between the lens and iris (posterior synechiae). These adhesions will block the flow of aqueous between the posterior and anterior chambers and result in forward ballooning of the iris and a rise in the intraocular pressure. Adhesions may also develop between the iris and cornea (peripheral anterior synechiae) covering up the trabecular drainage meshwork. Inflammatory cells may also block the meshwork. Topical steroids may cause a gradual asymptomatic rise in intraocular pressure that may lead to blindness. (Patients taking topical steroids over a long period should always be under ophthalmological supervision).

The growth of new vessels onto the iris (rubeosis) occurs both in diabetics and after occlusion of the central retinal vein as a consequence of retinal ischaemia. These vessels also block the trabecular meshwork, causing rubeotic glaucoma, which is extremely difficult to treat.

The trabecular meshwork itself may have developed abnormally (congenital glaucoma) or been damaged by trauma to the eye. Patients who have had eye injuries have a higher chance than normal of developing glaucoma later in life. If there is a bleed in the eye after trauma the red cells may also block the trabecular meshwork.

Medical treatment

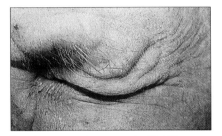

Eye closure to reduce systemic side effects after instilling drops.

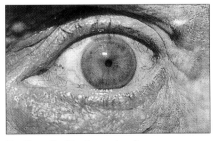

Small pupil with pilocarpine drops.

β blockers (e.g. timolol) — reduce the secretion of aqueous and are still the most commonly prescribed topical treatment. Contraindications to their use include a history of lung or heart disease, as the drops may cause systemic β blockade. Systemic effects from eyedrops can be reduced by occlusion of the punctum (finger pressed on the caruncle which can be felt as a lump at the inner canthus of the eye) or shutting the eyes for several minutes after putting in the drops. This reduces the lacrimal pumping mechanism, and stops the eyedrops running down the lacrimal passages and being absorbed systemically via the nasal mucosa, or by inhalation directly into the lungs. This may also enhance ocular absorption of the drugs.

Parasympathomimetic agents (e.g. pilocarpine) — constrict the pupil and "pull" on the trabecular meshwork, increasing the flow of the aqueous out of the eye. The small pupil may, however, cause visual problems if central lens opacities are present. Constriction of the ciliary body causes accommodation and blurred vision in young patients. Pilocarpine should not be used if there is inflammation in the eye as the pupil may stick to the lens close to the visual axis (posterior synechiae) and affect vision. Pilocarpine is usually administered four times a day but can be used twice in a combined form with a β blocker, or once in a gel preparation at night which reduces side effects.

Sympathomimetic agents — Topical adrenaline, once commonly prescribed, is now rarely used because of lack of efficacy with β blockers and adverse effects on the conjunctiva. A newer generation of agents that stimulate the α receptors of the sympathetic system is now used — for example bromonidine, used twice a day. Contraindications include cardiovascular disease, because of the potential systemic sympathomimetic effects.

Prostaglandin analogues (e.g. latanoprost) — This agent reduces the intraocular pressure by increasing aqueous outflow from the eye via an alternative drainage route called the uveoscleral pathway. Systemic side effects are minimal but an unusual side effect in a few patients with light irides is a permanent darkening of the iris.

Carbonic anhydrase inhibitors — are available as topical (e.g. dorzolamide) or oral (e.g. acetazolamide) agents. They reduce the secretion of aqueous, and the systemic, orally administered, form is the most powerful agent used to

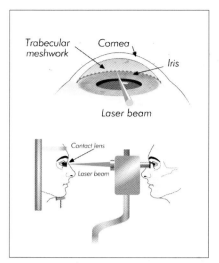

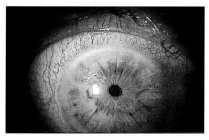

Laser trabeculoplasty.

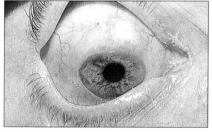

Hole made in the iris (iridotomy) with the neodymium-YAG laser without having to cut into the eyeball.

Conjunctival bleb after drainage operation.

reduce the intraocular pressure. Unfortunately, this may have many side effects, including nausea, lassitude, parasthesiae, and renal stones. The topical form has minimal side effects but is not as effective.

Laser treatment

Laser trabeculoplasty — Argon or diode laser "burns" are applied to the trabecular meshwork. How this treatment works is uncertain. It was thought to work by contracting one part of the meshwork, so stretching and opening up adjacent areas, but more recently it has been postulated that it rejuvenates the cells in the trabecular meshwork. This treatment is used only in the types of glaucoma where the drainage angle is open. The pressure-lowering effect is relatively short term, so this treatment is mainly used for more elderly patients.

Laser iridotomy — can be performed in cases of angle closure glaucoma with the Nd-YAG laser, which (unlike the argon or diode lasers) actually cuts holes in tissue rather than just burning. This procedure can be performed without incising the eye.

Laser ciliary body ablation — Lasers can be used to burn the circular ciliary body which produces aqueous humour. If a suitable wavelength is used the laser radiation can pass through the white sclera without being absorbed and only gets absorbed by the pigmented ciliary body (transcleral ciliary body photoablation). This treatment usually has to be repeated to maintain lowering of pressure and patients need to continue medical therapy.

Surgical treatment

Iridectomy — is performed in cases of angle closure glaucoma both in the affected eye and prophylactically in the other eye. Most of these cases can now be treated with the Nd-YAG laser.

Drainage surgery — A channel is created between the inside of the eye and the subconjunctival space, thus bypassing the blocked trabecular meshwork. A drainage "bleb" (aqueous under the conjunctiva) can often be seen under the upper lid. Conjunctivitis in a patient with a drainage bleb should always be treated promptly, as there is an increased risk of the infection entering the eye (endophthalmitis).

Surgery used to be resorted to only when medical treatment had failed to halt the progress of the disease, but is now being performed much earlier. The main cause of surgical failure is postoperative scarring leading to blockage of the new channel. The amount of scarring can now be reduced using anti-cancer agents. These are delivered by short applications during surgery on a sponge or by postoperative injections. The most commonly used drugs are 5-fluorouracil (5-FU) and mitomycin-c (MMC). There is an increased incidence of cataracts after drainage operations. In severe cases a drainage tube attached to a plastic plate, which acts as a drainage reservoir, can also be inserted.

9 Gradual visual loss, partial sight, and "blindness"

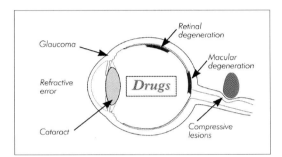

Causes of gradual visual loss.

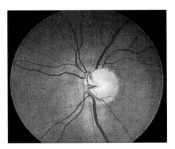

Cataracts.

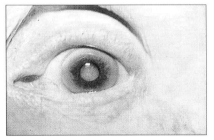

Glaucomatous cupping.

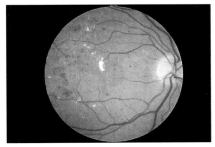

Background retinopathy with macular changes and good vision: refer.

Causes of gradual visual loss

Refractive errors — The pinhole test is a most useful test for identifying refractive errors. If there is a refractive error, the vision will improve. If the patient has thick glasses the pinhole should be used with the patient wearing them. After exclusion of other causes of visual loss, the patient can be sent to an optometrist for refraction and correction of refractive error (e.g. spectacles).

Corneal disease — Various disorders can cause gradual loss of the corneal endothelial cells and increasing oedema of the cornea. This leads to a gradual decrease in visual acuity which does not improve significantly with a pinhole. If the damage is advanced the cornea may appear opaque. A corneal graft from a donor may be required.

Cataract — This is probably the most common cause of gradual visual loss and the diagnosis may be made on viewing the red reflex. The patient should be referred if the visual disturbance interferes appreciably with the patient's lifestyle. If a patient with a cataract cannot project light or has an afferent pupillary defect, however, other diseases such as a retinal detachment must be excluded.

Primary open angle glaucoma — Unfortunately, the patient may not complain of visual disturbance until late in the course of the disease, hence the need for screening. Primary open angle glaucoma should, however, be excluded in any patient complaining of gradual visual loss. Any family history of glaucoma should be elicited. The vision may still be 6/6 so the visual field should be checked with a red pin, and cupping of, or asymmetry between, the optic discs should be sought.

Age related macular degeneration — This may occur gradually and is typified by loss of the central field. There are usually pigmentary changes at the macula. The disease occurs in both eyes, but it may be asymmetrical, and it is more common in shortsighted people. The gradual deterioration is not treatable, but if acute visual distortion supervenes during the course of the disease there may be a leaking area under the retina that can be treated with a laser.

Diabetic maculopathy — Diabetic retinopathy occurs in both insulin dependent and non-insulin dependent diabetics and affects all age groups. The patient may or may not give a history of diabetes, although the longer the duration of the diabetes, the more likely the patient is to have retinopathy. Background diabetic retinopathy is typified by microaneurysms, dot haemorrhages, and hard yellow exudates with well defined edges. Oedema of the macula may also be present and responsible for the fall in visual acuity, but this is less easily identified. This type of retinopathy at the macula (diabetic maculopathy) is the major cause of blindness in maturity onset diabetes, but it also occurs in younger, insulin dependent diabetics. It may be amenable to focal laser photocoagulation.

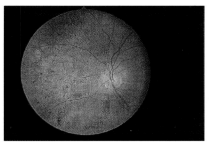

Retinitis pigmentosa: pigmentation and attenuated vessels.

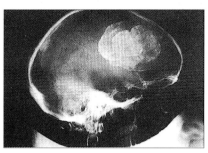

Radiograph showing calcified meningioma. Note that a plain skull radiograph will not show most intracranial tumours.

Aids to maximise low vision.

- Strong light from behind for reading
- Magnifying aids
- Large print books
- Closed circuit television

Helpful organisations.

Action for Blind People
14–16 Verney Road, London SE16 3DZ
Tel: 0171 732 8771
Provides information and advisory service for visually impaired people including benefits, grants and employment.

Action for Sick Children
Argyle House, 29–31 Euston Road
London NW1 2SD
Tel: 0171 833 2041
Supports families of sick children and works to ensure effective planning of health services for sick children.

Benefits Agency Helpline
Tel: 0800 882200 (freephone)
Advice on benefits.

Contact a Family
170 Tottenham Court Road, London W1P 0HA
Contactline 0171 383 3555 (national helpline)
Provides services at national, regional and local levels for parents and professionals, and a directory of specific conditions and rare syndromes.

Hereditary degeneration of the retina — These conditions are relatively rare but should be suspected if there is a family history of visual deterioration. Symptoms include night blindness and intolerance to light. Most types of retinal degeneration are not yet treatable, but some are associated with metabolic disorders that can be treated. These patients need to be referred to an ophthalmologist, preferably one with a special interest in these conditions, for diagnosis and any possible treatments.

Patients with severe visual impairment may develop visual hallucinations and sleep disturbance. It is particularly important for these patients to have an opportunity to discuss the diagnosis, prognosis and genetic counselling. Much can be done to help patients through psychosocial counselling (see below, Management of gradual visual loss).

Compressive lesions of the optic pathways — These are relatively rare, but should always be considered. The history and examination may give clues if there are headaches, focal neurological signs or endocrinological abnormalities such as acromegaly. There should not be an afferent pupillary defect in most patients with cataract, macular degeneration or refractive error. Testing of the visual fields may show the bitemporal field defect of a pituitary tumour. The discs should be checked for optic atrophy and papilloedema.

Drugs — Several drugs may cause visual loss. In particular, a history of excessive alcohol intake or smoking, methanol ingestion, or the taking of chloroquine or ethambutol should lead to the suspicion of drug induced visual deterioration. Systemic or topical steroids may cause cataracts and glaucoma.

Management of gradual visual loss

The initial management of gradual visual loss depends on the cause. Refractive errors usually require no more than a pair of spectacles. Cataracts can be removed and an artificial lens implanted. Glaucoma requires treatment to lower the intraocular pressure. Patients with unexplained visual loss should always be referred.

There are, however, a significant number of conditions that are not amenable to medical or surgical treatment. Despite this, there is still much that can be done for the patient.

Good lighting. The patient should be advised to use adequate lighting. Using a brighter light bulb may make all the difference. Patients should be advised to read with a strong light placed behind them. This reduces glare, maximises contrast between the print and the page and may reduce excessive pupillary constriction that would otherwise impair vision, especially if the patient has cataracts. A booklet called *Lighting and Low Vision* is available from the Partially Sighted Society (see addresses below).

Low vision aids. A simple magnifying glass may be a great help. Books with large print are available from most public libraries. There are also special magnifying aids that can be attached to spectacles; these differ from a simple magnifying glass in that they allow magnification without the patient having to get extremely close to the print. Many eye departments have a low vision aids service that is usually run by an optometrist. It may be possible to obtain such aids on loan from the departments. Closed circuit television can be used to magnify text and may allow a visually disabled person to do a "normal" job. Various home aids are also available such as tactile markings for cookers. Details are available from the local electricity and gas suppliers in conjunction with the Royal National Institute for the Blind (RNIB).

Psychosocial support. There is a strong need for psychosocial support following a diagnosis of a blinding disorder, and at subsequent stages of sight loss. Some specialised eye departments provide this help as part of a

Helpful organisations (continued).

Disability Law Service
Room 241, 2nd Floor, 49–51 Bedford Row,
London WC1R 4LR
Tel: 0171 831 8031
Provides legal advice on issues such as employment, driving, and benefits.

Guide Dogs for the Blind Association
Hillfields, Burghfield Common, Reading
Berkshire RG7 3YG
Tel: 01734 835555
Provides guide dogs for partially sighted and blind people. They have also extended their service by offering long cane training and rehabilitation for daily living.

Local Social Services and Education Authorities
Addresses in the local telephone directory or from Citizens Advice Bureaux. May run child-minding service, provide home helps or provide creches or day nurseries.

LOOK
Queen Alexandra College, 49 Court Oak Road
Harborne, Birmingham B17 9TG
Tel: 0121 428 5038
LOOK is a national organisation pledged to help and support families throughout the United Kingdom to enable them to speak with one voice and to help secure appropriate provision for the health, welfare and education of children.

LOOK (Scotland)
Answerphone 0131 313 5711

Partially Sighted Society
PO Box 322, Doncaster DN1 2XA
Tel: 01302 323132
Contact main office in Doncaster for local self-help branches. Provision of equipment and advice on living and working with impaired vision.

RLSB (Royal London Society for the Blind)
Head Office: Dorton House School, Seal
Near Sevenoaks, Kent TN15 0ED
Tel: 01732 592500
The RLSB provides a comprehensive service for children and adults with visual impairment. This includes advocacy, counselling, education, further education, rehabilitation, training for work and job placement.
For further information, contact the RLSB Information Officer, Dorton Training Services
Tel: 0181 782 7800.
Web site: <http:\\www.rlsb.org.uk>

RNIB (Royal National Institute for the Blind)
224 Great Portland Street, London W1N 6AA
Tel: 0171 388 1266
Offers a comprehensive range of services for visually impaired people covering benefits, education and health information. Practical equipment can be purchased from the RNIB's Customer Service department based in Peterborough; tel: 0345 023153.

SENSE
11–13 Clifton Terrace, Finsbury Park
London N4 3SR
Tel: 0171 272 7774
SENSE is a national voluntary organisation supporting and campaigning for people who are deaf, deaf–blind, their families, carers and professionals who work with them. Available to people of all ages and widely varying conditions.

INTERNET
Further information about several of these support groups is available on the Internet.

multidisciplinary team. However, the vast majority of patients may only receive this help via their local authority Social Service Department or possibly a voluntary society for the visually impaired. The diagnosis of a disease causing significant visual disability can be devastating for patients, particularly for the parents of children with these conditions.

A summary of guidelines, and more detailed guidelines for professionals involved with newly-diagnosed blind and partially sighted children and their families can be obtained free from the RNIB (see addresses below).

Registration as partially sighted or blind. This confers various benefits, which are shown below. The patient has to be referred to a consultant ophthalmologist who, with the patient's agreement, completes a form (BD8). The requirements for registration are:

Partially sighted — The patient must have vision of 6/60 or worse in both eyes. The vision can be better than 6/60 if the visual fields are markedly reduced; for example, a patient with 6/6 vision but severely restricted fields caused by primary open angle glaucoma. A patient who has an homonymous hemianopia following a stroke should be offered the option of being registered partially sighted.

Blind — The current statutory definition of blindness is "that a person should be so blind as to be unable to perform any work for which eyesight is essential". The guidelines for registration as blind are a visual acuity of 3/60 or worse in both eyes. Again, the visual acuity can be better than this if the visual fields are abnormal.

These criteria are flexible and the final decision is left to the consultant ophthalmologist who will take other ocular problems into consideration. It is important that the patient does not feel that all hope is lost and that eventually everything will go completely "dark". This is particularly the case for patients with age related macular degeneration in which only central vision is lost. In this case the patient can be told that he will not go blind because he will still have peripheral vision. A patient with vision of counting fingers may still be virtually independent within the home, despite being registered as blind. Therefore it is very important to emphasise to patients that blind registration does not mean total blindness in the lay sense of the word.

Blind or partial sight registration is not essential but is helpful when accessing financial benefits and specialist support and advice from local authorities. Once the local authority social service department has received the registration form, a number of support services should then be available to the visually impaired person. Each local authority keeps a register of blind and partially sighted people living within the area. The social worker is the key person to contact, but a visually impaired person may need a range of support services.

Special education and training. Advice about mainstream and special schools for visually impaired children can be obtained from local education authorities. Help and advice for parents, particularly about their child's placement and their right of appeal, is offered by the Royal National Institute for the Blind and the Royal London Society for the Blind advocacy service for parents. The needs of each child can be assessed by the local education authority in order to provide the appropriate educational support. This may be in mainstream schools, or schools for visually impaired children. In some cases, this may lead to a statement of special educational needs.

Employment and training. Information and advice is available from the RNIB Employment Network, the Disability Employment Adviser of the local job centre (Employment Services), Action for Blind People and the Royal London Society for the Blind. Practical support, such as modification to equipment and help with fares to and from work, can be accessed through the Disability Employment Adviser of the local job centre.

Gradual visual loss, partial sight, and "blindness"

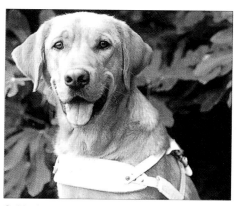
Guide dog.

Mobility and technical training. Rehabilitation officers are employed by local authorities to teach a whole range of skills, such as Braille, mobility skills, and daily living skills. In some parts of the country, this work is undertaken by staff from the Guide Dogs for the Blind Association, and/or the local voluntary organisation for the visually impaired.

Self-help support groups and other organisations. Visually impaired people and their families need advice, practical help and information, both at the time of diagnosis and at subsequent stages of sight loss. These can be provided by support groups and other organisations. The boxes here contain many useful addresses and telephone numbers.

Genetic counselling. Patients with hereditary visual problems should have the opportunity to discuss the implications with a geneticist. Most regions have a genetic counselling service.

Useful publications, media and services.

Guidelines for health professionals
Summary guidelines for good practice for health professionals involved with newly diagnosed blind or partially sighted children and their families are available:

● Summary guidelines (leaflet) — *Taking the Time: telling parents their child is blind or partially sighted* can be obtained free from:
RNIB Children's Policy Unit, 24 Great Portland Street, London W1N 6AA; tel: 0171 388 1266

● More detailed guidelines (book) — *Taking the Time: telling parents their child is blind or partially sighted* compiled with parents and representatives of more than 20 professional organisations is available from:
RNIB Customer Services, PO Box 173, Peterborough PE2 6WS; tel: 0345 023153
Price £10.00; please quote code PR11005.

Talking newspapers and talking books
There are a wide variety of taped services available nationally and locally, some examples of which are given below. All the services below are dispatched under the "Articles for the blind" Freepost service.

Calibre
Aylesbury, Bucks HP22 5XQ
Tel: 01296 432339
Talking books on standard audio cassettes for visually impaired children and adults.

Royal London Society for the Blind
RLSB Industrial Services
Unit 1, Ursula Lapp Estate
1 Old Oak Lane
Park Royal
London NW10 6UD
Tel: 0181 838 4384
Fax: 0181 838 4417
Books recorded on standard audio cassettes.

Talking Newspapers Association of the UK (TNAUK)
90 High Street, Heathfield
East Sussex TN21 8JO
Tel: 01435 866102
More than 150 titles of national newspapers and magazines provided on standard audio cassettes.

RNIB Talking Book Service
Mount Pleasant, Wembley
Middlesex HA0 1RR
Tel: 0181 903 6666
Taped book service requiring special machine with easy-to-operate controls.

RNIB Cassette Library
PO Box 173
Peterborough PE2 6WS
Tel: 0345 023153
Wide range of titles, including academic subjects, recorded on standard standard audio cassettes.

Languages other than English
A growing number of titles are now available in other languages such as Welsh, Gaelic, Hindi, Urdu, Gujerati and Bengali. Details of these and other tape services can be obtained from RNIB Customer Services on 0345 023153.

Large print books
These can be borrowed from most public libraries and the RNIB.
For a list of books to buy, including titles for children and visually imparied parents wishing to teach their sighted child, please contact RNIB Customer Services, 0345 023153. Books can also be purchased from:

Chivers Press Publishers
Windsor Bridge Road, Bath BA2 3AX
Tel: 01225 335336

ISIS
55 St Thomas's Street, Oxford OX1 1JG
Tel: 01865 250333

Magna
Magna House, Long Preston
Near Skipton, North Yorkshire BD23 4ND
Tel: 01729 840225

Ulverscroft
The Green, Bradgate Road
Anstey, Leicester LE7 7FU
Tel: 0116 2364325

CD ROMs
CD ROMs have opened up new possibilities for visually impaired children and adults. References can be swiftly found and read immediately though the braille, speech or large character display output of a computer. Students can do their own research or browse at will. *Opening up the library for visually impaired learners* gives details. Free copies from the RNIB Education Centre, London.
Tel: 0171 388 1266.

Radio programme
In Touch
A radio programme is broadcast weekly on BBC Radio 4 and reports on issues that affect the lives of visually impaired people in the United Kingdom.

Specialist centres
In most towns, there are specialist centres where blind and partially sighted people can obtain information, examine and sometimes buy equipment suited to their needs. The facilities that centres provide vary widely. They are mainly run by local voluntary societies for the visually impaired.

10　Squint

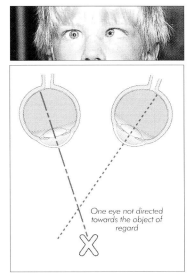

The true definition of squint.

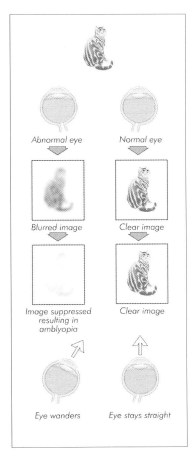

A squint may be a sign of impaired visual acuity.

The subject of squint (strabismus) is one that many practitioners approach with great trepidation, sometimes with justification. If, however, it is approached systematically much of the myth and mystery can be dispelled.

What is a squint?

The word is used in many different ways. It is often used to describe the narrowing of the gap between the upper and lower eyelids (interpalpebral fissure), usually carried out by patients to create a pinhole effect. This reduces the consequences of any refractive error, and improves the clarity of the image. The true definition of squint, however, is that one of the eyes is not directed towards the object under scrutiny. It should be noted that when the eyes converge for close work there is no squint.

Why is a squint important?

A squint may show that the acuity of the eye is impaired because of ocular disease. The eyes are kept straight by the drive to keep the image of the object being viewed in the centre of the macular area, where highest definition and colour vision is located. The tone in the extraocular muscles is constantly being readjusted to maintain this fixation. If the vision is impaired in one or both eyes this constant readjustment cannot occur and one eye may wander.

This is important, as the cause of impaired vision may be eminently treatable, as in the case of a cataract or a refractive error. It is especially important in a child because, unlike that of an adult, a child's vision may be irreversibly impaired if treatment is not given in time. The visual pathways in the brain receiving information from an abnormal eye fail to develop normally. The resulting depressed cortical function leads to amblyopia, commonly called a "lazy" eye. It is important to realise that a child does not complain that the sight of one eye is poor, and the prevention of a permanent impaired acuity may require no more than a pair of spectacles to correct a refractive error.

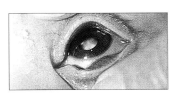

Congenital cataract.

A squint may itself cause amblyopia in a child — Misalignment of the eyes may be the primary problem, with resulting double vision. Young children do not normally complain of double vision. In a young child the vision of one eye may be suppressed to avoid this diplopia and the visual pathways then fail to develop properly. This leads to amblyopia of the eye that is otherwise organically sound.

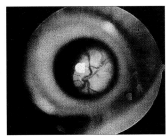

Retinoblastoma in a child presenting with a squint.

A squint may be a sign of a life threatening condition — Squint is a common presentation in a child with a retinoblastoma. The resulting squint is non-paralytic and therefore the angle of deviation is the same irrespective of the direction of gaze. The eye deviates

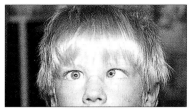

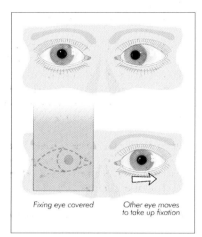

Left convergent squint: note position of light reflexes.

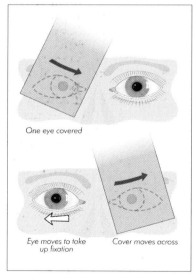

Cover/uncover test.

Alternate cover test.

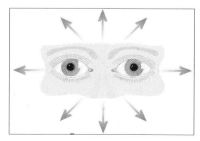

Test eye movements in all directions of gaze.

because vision is impaired and this may occur in any eye with visual impairment. A squint can also be caused by a sixth nerve palsy resulting from a tumour that is causing raised intracranial pressure. In this case the squint will be paralytic and the angle of squint will vary depending on the direction of gaze. Patients with myasthenia gravis may present with a squint and diplopia.

How can a squint be detected and assessed clinically?

Adults may complain of deviation of the eyes or of diplopia. Children are brought because their parents or other relatives notice either one or both eyes turning in or out, or there may be a family history of squint. Children may also be referred from vision screening clinics.

History
A family history of squint is a strong risk factor in the development of squint, and if there is any doubt the child should be referred. Children with disorders of the central nervous system such as cerebral palsy have a higher incidence of squint than normal children. Problems during birth and retarded development also increase the likelihood of a squint. The parents' visual problems should be ascertained, particularly large refractive errors.

The earlier the age of onset the more likely is the need for an operation. A constant squint has a worse visual prognosis than one that is intermittent.

Examination
Check the visual acuity — If the visual acuity does not correct with spectacles or a pinhole, ocular disease or amblyopia must be suspected. This is particularly important in children as the amblyopia or ocular problems must be treated immediately if sight is to be preserved. Visual acuity in infants is difficult to assess. A history from the mother is useful to find out whether the baby looks at her and at objects. If, however, only one eye is affected the visual problem may not be apparent. If the sight is poor in only one eye, covering the good eye may make the child try to push the cover away. In an older child small coloured sweets may be used to get a rough estimate of the acuity. The older child may also be able to match letters.

Look at the position of the patient's eyes — Large squints will be obvious. Wide epicanthic folds may give the impression of a squint (pseudosquint), but children with wide epicanthic folds may still have true squints.

Look at the corneal reflections of a bright light held in front of the eyes — Note the position of the reflections; they should be symmetrical. This test gives a rough estimate of the angle of any deviation.

Cover test — There are two types of cover tests that help to reveal a squint, especially if it is small and the examiner is unsure about the position of the corneal reflections. In the cover/uncover test one eye is covered and the other eye is observed. If the uncovered eye moves to fix on the object there is a squint that is present all the time — a manifest squint. The test should then be carried out on the other eye. A problem arises when the vision in the squinting eye is reduced, and the eye may not be able to take up fixation. This emphasises the need to test the vision of any patient with squint. If the cover/uncover test is normal (indicating no manifest squint) the alternate cover test should be done. In this test the occluder is moved to and fro between the eyes. If the eye that has been uncovered moves, then there is a latent squint.

Test eye movements in all directions of gaze — If there is a paralytic squint, the degree of deviation will vary with the direction of gaze. An adult will often say that the separation of the images varies, and increases in the direction of action of the weakened muscles.

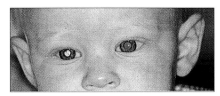

White reflex of retinoblastoma.

Examination of the eye with a pupil dilating agent (mydriatic) and a ciliary muscle relaxing agent (cycloplegic) — Any overt abnormalities of the eye should be noted. The reasons for dilating the pupil is to exclude retinal disease such as a retinoblastoma, and the cycloplegic allows a check for any refractive error. Adequate examination of the peripheral fundus and refraction require dilation of the pupil and special equipment. Nevertheless, cataracts and other opacities in the media, and the white reflex that is suggestive of retinoblastoma, may readily be checked for by looking at the red reflex without dilating the pupil.

Management

Paralytic squints usually occur in adults. Underlying conditions such as raised intracranial pressure, compressive lesions, and diseases such as diabetes, hypertension, myasthenia gravis and dysthyroid eye disease should be excluded.

If diplopia is a problem one eye may need to be occluded temporarily, for example, by a patch stuck to the patient's spectacles. Alternatively, temporary prisms may be stuck onto the spectacles to eliminate the diplopia. An operation on the ocular muscles may be indicated if the squint stabilises. If an operation on the muscles is either inappropriate or proves inadequate, permanent prisms may be incorporated into the spectacle prescription.

Non-paralytic squints usually occur in children. If the squint is caused by disease in the eye that is itself causing reduced vision and subsequent deviation of the eye (for example, cataract) this needs to be treated. Types of treatment for non-paralytic squints are described below.

Spectacles — There are two main indications for prescribing spectacles in children.

Firstly, spectacles should be given to the child who is hypermetropic (longsighted) and has a convergent squint. Normally when the ciliary muscle contracts the lens becomes more globular to allow the eye to focus on close objects (accommodation). This is linked to convergence so that both eyes can fix on the close object.

If the child is hypermetropic the ciliary muscle has to contract strongly for the child to be able to focus on a near object. This excessive accommodation may cause overconvergence so that a squint occurs. This type of aquint is termed an accommodative

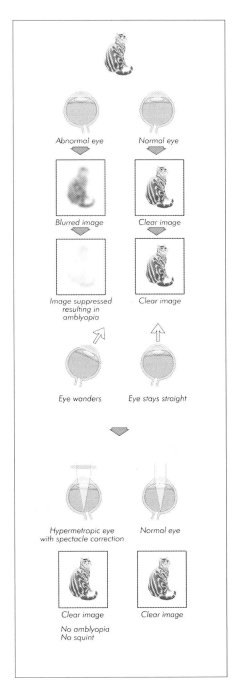

Amblyopia and squint caused by refractive error, and the use of spectacles to treat the refractive error and prevent amblyopia.

The use of spectacles to treat an accomodative convergent squint in a long sighted child.

convergent squint. The use of hypermetropic glasses in this case relaxes the ciliary muscles and removes the drive to overconverge.

Secondly, spectacles are prescribed for the child who has a refractive error, particularly if this is unilateral. As a consequence of the refractive error the image on the retina will be indistinct. The visual pathways will then not develop properly (resulting in amblyopia). Children with a refractive error may not develop a squint until the vision is poor in one eye, which emphasises the need to check the visual acuity. The use of spectacles may therefore prevent a child from developing severe visual loss in an otherwise "normal" eye — hence the need to refract every child with a squint or impaired vision.

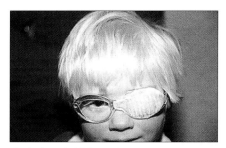

Occlusion of child's good eye to stimulate amblyopic eye.

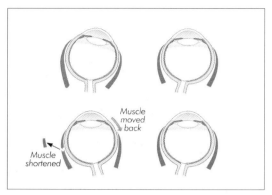

Operation for squint.

Occlusion. This is the well known patching of one eye to encourage the development of the visual pathway of the "bad" eye. If the development of one pathway has been retarded by a squint or refractive error this pathway can be stimulated if the "good" eye is patched. This can, however, only be done for a limited period, and there is a danger of the good eye itself becoming amblyopic. The underlying problem must, of course, be corrected in the meantime. The vision of the good eye may also be "blurred" with drops such as atropine.

Orthoptic treatment — A series of visual exercises may encourage the simultaneous use of both eyes.

Operation — The ocular muscles can be repositioned to straighten the eyes. Spectacles are prescribed and occlusion performed before operation because an eye is more likely to stay straight if the vision is good. In adults "adjustable" surgery can be carried out. The muscle position is adjusted by altering the tension on the sutures postoperatively.

Botulinum toxin — Very small amounts of botulinum toxin can be injected into overacting muscles. This paralyses the muscles for a few months and this treatment can be repeated. It can also permit the assessment of the effect of prospective surgery before permanent surgery is carried out.

In the older child — The effectiveness of treatment in reversing amblyopia decreases as the child gets older. Once the child is about 8 or 9 years old the visual system is no longer flexible and amblyopia cannot be reversed. The child may, however, still need glasses to correct any refractive error, and an operation may be required if the squint poses a cosmetic problem.

11 General medical disorders and the eye

Systemic diseases with ocular manifestations.

- Diabetes mellitus
- Hypertension
- Dysthyroid eye disease
- Rheumatoid arthritis
- Other arthritides
- Rosacea
- Sarcoid
- Congenital rubella
- AIDS

Few serious medical conditions do not affect the eye. It is important to know the ocular manifestations of systemic diseases for several reasons.

- *Screening is required to detect early ocular changes that may require treatment to prevent blindness.* A good example is a diabetic patient with new vessels on the optic disc, which signal an exceptionally high risk of visual loss unless treatment is given in time.
- *Knowledge of the ocular complications of other diseases may help in the diagnosis of an ocular problem.* A red, locally injected, and tender eye in a patient with rheumatoid arthritis suggests scleritis, which may progress to perforation of the eye. Iritis should be strongly considered in a young man with ankylosing spondylitis who presents with a red eye.
- *The ocular symptoms may suggest the systemic disease* (for example, prominent eyes and lid lag in hyperthyroidism) *or confirm it* (for example, the Kayser-Fleisher ring of copper in Wilson's disease).
- *The ocular signs may have prognostic value.* If cotton wool spots occur in the eyes of an otherwise asymptomatic patient with AIDS the prognosis is particularly poor.

Diabetes mellitus

Diabetes mellitus is the commonest cause of blindness among people of working age in the Western world. Two percent of the diabetic population are blind, many of them in the younger age groups. Much of this eye disease can be treated, which makes early identification and referral crucial.

What are the treatable causes of visual loss in diabetics, and how can they be detected early enough to be effectively treated?

Cataract and primary open angle glaucoma are more common in diabetic than in non-diabetic patients. Cataract can be treated by surgical removal, and primary open angle glaucoma can be treated by drugs and operations that lower the intraocular pressure. Cataract and glaucoma can often be detected by viewing the red reflex and examining the optic disc, respectively. It is only too easy to forget to look for glaucomatous cupping of the disc when looking for the signs of diabetic retinopathy.

Blinding diabetic retinopathy occurs in both insulin dependent and non-insulin dependent diabetic patients and affects all age groups. The longer the duration of the diabetes, the more likely the patient is to have retinopathy (about 80% are affected after 20 years). Again this applies to all categories of diabetic patients. However, the better the control of blood sugar levels the lower the incidence of diabetic retinopathy. Patients with diabetes should have their pupils dilated yearly with tropicamide 1% and the fundi examined if important physical signs are not to be missed. There are two main clinical types of retinopathy that cause blindness in diabetics, and these need to be identified and the patients referred for early treatment.

Background retinopathy — typified by microaneurysms, dot haemorrhages, and hard yellow exudates with well defined edges. These changes do not have much affect on vision when they occur in the peripheral retina. When they occur in the macula area, however, central vision may be severely

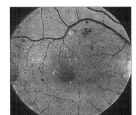

Background retinopathy: hard exudates, microaneurysms, and haemorrhages.

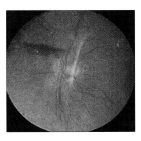

Proliferative retinopathy: new vessels, fibrosis, and haemorrhage.

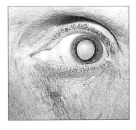

Cataract in a diabetic patient.

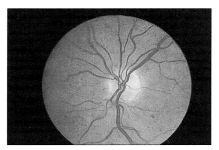

Background retinopathy with good acuity: review regularly.

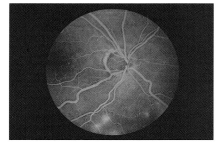

Fluorescein angiogram showing areas of leakage.

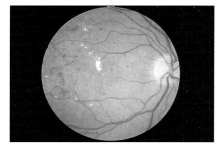

Background retinopathy with macular changes and good vision: refer.

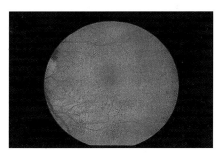

Background retinopathy with impaired acuity: refer.

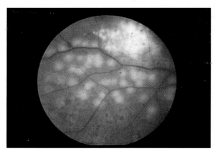

Diabetic retinopathy: recent and old laser burns.

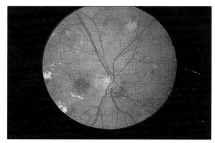

Preproliferative retinopathy. Cotton wool spots, large haemorrhages, and tortuous veins: refer urgently.

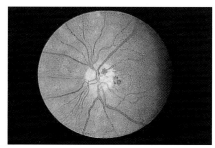

Proliferative retinopathy: refer immediately.

affected. Backgound retinopathy at the macula (diabetic maculopathy) is the major cause of blindness in maturity onset diabetes, but it also occurs in younger, insulin dependent diabetics. It may be amenable to focal laser photocoagulation, which may help to reduce any leakage. This is particularly true when hard exudates are a prominent feature of the maculopathy.

Proliferative retinopathy — typified by the growth of new vessels on the retina or into the vitreous cavity. This is thought to result from the ischaemic diabetic retina producing vasoproliferative factors that cause the growth of abnormal new vessels. These vessels may bleed causing a sudden decrease in vision because of a vitreous haemorrhage. Worse still, this blood often results in the production of contractile membranes that gradually pull off the retina, causing blindness. This may occur in any diabetic patient, but more commonly in young, insulin dependent patients. The vision may be 6/6 right up to the moment of a bleed, hence the need for early detection of new vessels by adequate fundal examination. Fluorescein angiography may be necessary to help to identify areas of retinal ischaemia and new vessel formation. New vessels may also grow at the front of the eye onto the iris and occlude the drainage angle of the anterior chamber causing glaucoma (rubeotic glaucoma).

Laser treatment (or any other method of photocoagulation) is used to treat proliferative retinopathy. The laser, however, is not usually used to coagulate new vessels as these may bleed or recur. When a patient has new vessels at the disc, the entire retina is treated with laser, except for the macula area, which preserves the central vision. Hence, the term "panretinal photocoagulation" or "pattern bombing". This destroys much of the ischaemic peripheral retina and stops it producing the vasoproliferative factors that induce the growth of new vessels, and often the new vessels regress. New blood vessels on the iris that block the outflow of aqueous and cause rubeotic glaucoma may also regress. It may, however, require thousands of laser burns and repeated treatments to achieve this. This treatment may significantly reduce peripheral vision, and mean that the patient may have to give up driving.

Screening for diabetic eye disease
Patients may be divided into five groups for screening purposes.
- *Those with no retinopathy or with background retinopathy and normal vision when tested with glasses or pinhole.* These patients can be reviewed yearly with dilatation of the pupils. They should be told to attend sooner if there is a change in vision that is not corrected with glasses.
- *Those with background retinopathy and changes around the macula area.* They should be referred to an ophthalmologist as this may herald a blinding maculopathy.
- *Those with background retinopathy and impaired acuity not corrected with glasses or pinhole.* It may be that the patient has an oedematous or ischaemic form of maculopathy that is extremely hard to diagnose with the direct ophthalmoscope alone. The oedematous form may respond to focal laser treatment if this is given early.
- *Those with preproliferative retinopathy.* They have no new vessels, but the haemorrhages are larger, the veins are tortuous, and there are cotton wool spots. These physical signs imply that the retina is ischaemic and that there is a high risk that new vessels will subsequently form. These patients should be referred.

Measures to improve prognosis in diabetic retinopathy.

- Control blood sugar
- Control hypertension
- Control hyperlipidaemia
- Stop smoking

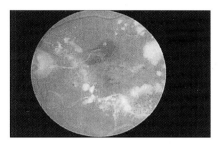

Retinopathy in accelerated hypertension with macular exudates and occluded vessels; disc swelling has resolved.

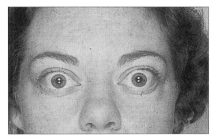

Hyperthyroidism with lid retraction.

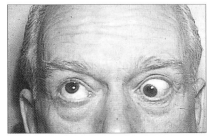

Autoimmune eye disease with restriction of ocular movements.

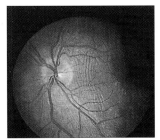

Choroidal folds.

- *Those with proliferative retinopathy.* This is typified by new blood vessels, and sometimes soft cotton wool spots, fibrosis, and vitreous haemorrhages. These patients need immediate referral, particularly if there are vitreous haemorrhages.

In addition to ocular treatment, blood sugar control should be carefully controlled. If the blood sugar concentration is brought under control rapidly, the fundus should be reviewed regularly during this period as there may be a transient worsening of the retinopathy. There is no question that good control of the blood sugar level reduces diabetic retinopathy. Hypertension and hyperlipidaemia worsen the prognosis of retinopathy and must also be controlled. Patients should be strongly advised not to smoke.

Diabetic individuals are also more prone to recurrent corneal abrasions, retinal vein occlusions and cranial nerve palsies. Aids for a diabetic with impaired vision include an audible click count syringe, and a Hypotest instrument that gives an audible signal with urinary Diastix.

Hypertension

The mild fundal changes of hypertension are extremely common. "Silver wiring" of the retinal arteries and arteriovenous nipping are well known signs, but arteriolar narrowing is the most reliable fundal sign.

Accelerated hypertension is classically associated with swelling of the head of the optic nerve. Any patient with hard exudates, cotton wool spots, or haemorrhages as a result of hypertension has a grave prognosis. Patients with these fundal signs should have their blood pressure checked and diabetes excluded. Urgent referral to a physician is required as this combination of signs may not only result in blindness but is also life threatening. Retinal vein occlusion is also more common in hypertensive patients.

Dysthyroid eye disease

Patients may have signs associated with hyperthyroidism and the consequent overaction of the sympathetic system. These patients have retracted upper and lower lids caused by excessive stimulation of sympathetically innervated muscles in the eyelids. This also gives rise to the well known sign of lid lag when the patient looks downwards. These features may suggest the diagnosis when the patient walks into the surgery.

If these signs are present, thyroid dysfunction should be excluded. If there are no visual problems, no corneal exposure, and the eyes move normally the patient need not be referred. Patients may, however, also have evidence of autoimmune disease directed against the orbital contents, particularly the muscles. These signs may be associated with the classic signs of Graves' disease, including goitre, pseudoclubbing of the fingers (thyroid acropathy), hyperthyroidism, and pretibial myxoedema. Autoimmune ocular disease may also occur on its own with no thyroid dysfunction. The clinical features include the following:

- *Swelling of the eyelids.*
- *Oedema (chemosis) and engorgement of the blood vessels of the conjunctiva.*
- *Exposure of the cornea* because of lack of blinking and failure of the lids to cover the eye adequately.
- *Pronounced protrusion of the eyes.* The absence of this feature in association with the other features may be even more serious as it may be that a tight orbital septum is holding back the swollen orbital contents. This may lead to a rise in intraocular pressure as well as pressure on the optic nerve.
- *Restriction of eye movements.* This is caused by infiltration of the muscles with inflammatory cells, and consequent inflammation, oedema and finally fibrosis.
- *Optic neuropathy.* This is relatively rare. The fundal signs include vascular congestion and swelling or atrophy of the head of the optic nerve. There may be "folds" in the choroid caused by pressure on the globe. This should be excluded in any patient with autoimmune eye disease who experiences visual deterioration.

These features may occur in any combination.

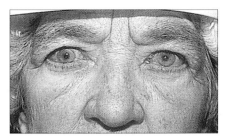
Patient with mild dysthyroid eye disease: red eyes and exposure as a result of infrequent blinking.

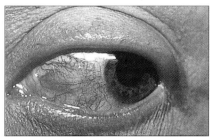
Episcleritis.

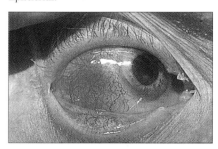
Scleritis.

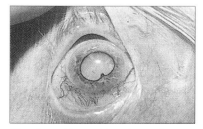
Chronic anterior uveitis and secondary cataract in seronegative arthritis.

Management of dysthyroid eye disease
- Associated thyroid dysfunction should be excluded, though treatment of any dysfunction may make no difference to the eye disease, and may even make it worse.
- Artificial tears should be used to lubricate the cornea and prevent drying and corneal ulceration.
- If there are cosmetic or exposure problems caused by lid retraction, guanethidine drops 5% may reduce the lid retraction by relaxing the sympathetically controlled retractor muscles. Occasionally an operation on these muscles may be required.
- If corneal exposure is threatening sight, the eyelids may have to be sewn together temporarily (tarsorrhaphy).
- Prisms incorporated in the patient's glasses may help to correct any double vision.
- Operations on the muscles of eye movement may be required to realign the eyes in patients with longstanding diplopia that has stabilized. Recently the introduction of local injections of minute doses of botulinum toxin to paralyse specific extraocular muscles has meant that patients with restrictive muscle diseases may sometimes be treated at an earlier stage.
- In serious disease with corneal problems or pressure on the optic nerve emergency treatment may be required, which may include high doses of steroids, surgical orbital compression, and radiotherapy. The visual fields may be restricted and there may be a relative afferent pupillary defect. Changes in colour vision, which may be noticed while watching colour television, may be an important sign of optic nerve compression, and patients should be told to inform their doctor immediately if these changes are noticed.

Rheumatoid arthritis

Rheumatoid arthritis is another common condition in which ocular complications are frequent. The lacrimal glands are also affected by an inflammatory process with consequent inadequate tear flow. The patient complains of dry, gritty and sore eyes. Treatment consists of replacement artificial tear drops instilled as often as necessary. Simple ointment may also help, but this will blur the vision if used during the day. If there is an aggregation of mucus, mucolytic eye drops (for example, acetylcysteine) may help, but patients should be warned that these sting.

The inflammatory process may also affect the episcleral and scleral coats of the eye causing the patient to complain of a red, uncomfortable eye. The redness is usually focal and there is tenderness over the area. Scleritis is usually much more painful than episcleritis and the engorged vessels are deeper. If scleritis continues the sclera may become thin (scleromalacia) and the eye may eventually perforate (scleromalacia perforans). The patient should be referred, as systemic treatment may be indicated.

These processes may also occur in other connective tissue diseases such as systemic lupus erythematosus, scleroderma, and dermatomyositis.

Other arthritides

The seronegative arthritides include ankylosing spondylitis, Reiter's syndrome, psoriatic arthritis and arthritis associated with inflammatory bowel disease. Acute anterior uveitis (iritis, iridocyclitis) is much more common in these patients. If a patient with any of these conditions has a red eye, anterior uveitis should be suspected. This is particularly true if the patient has had past attacks, and "experienced" patients often know when an attack is coming on. The patient should be referred for early treatment, which may prevent some of the complications of anterior uveitis.

Seronegative childhood arthritis is a particularly important cause of chronic anterior uveitis. The great danger is that the eyes in this condition are often white and pain-free, and the child may not complain of any visual problems. There may be secondary cataracts that may cause

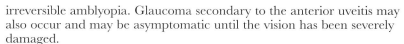

Risk factors for ocular involvement in childhood seronegative arthritis.

- Female sex
- Fewer than five joints affected
- Antinuclear antibodies

irreversible amblyopia. Glaucoma secondary to the anterior uveitis may also occur and may be asymptomatic until the vision has been severely damaged.

The group of children particularly at risk are females, those with fewer than five joints affected by the arthritis (pauciarticular), and those with antinuclear antibodies in their blood. These children should be referred to an ophthalmologist.

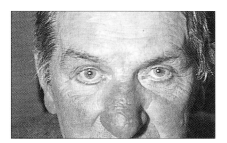

Rosacea and associated blepharitis.

Rosacea

Rosacea may seriously affect the eyes. There is often associated blepharitis, which may result in recurrent chalazia and styes. The abnormal lids and lipid secretion affect the tear film and the symptoms of "dry eye" result. The cornea scars, particularly in the inferonasal and inferotemporal areas, with neovascularization. Thinning occurs and the cornea may occasionally perforate.

Treatment with tear substitutes is indicated together with treatment for any associated blepharitis. Systemic tetracycline (250 mg four times daily for up to a month, then daily for several months) may considerably improve the patient's ocular as well as facial condition.

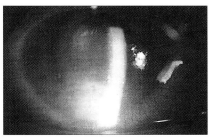

Anterior uveitis in sarcoidosis: large deposits of inflammatory white cells on posterior surface of cornea.

Sarcoid

Sarcoid is associated with various ocular problems. Acute uveitis and chronic uveitis occur, which may result in cataract, glaucoma, and a band of calcium deposited in the cornea (band keratopathy). The lacrimal glands may be infiltrated resulting in symptoms of "dry eye" requiring tear replacement. The granulomatous process may also affect the posterior part of the eye in the form of vasculitis and sometimes infiltration of the optic nerve.

Ocular manifestations of congenital rubella.

- Cataract
- Squint
- Refractive error
- Glaucoma
- Retinopathy

Congenital rubella

The ocular manifestations of congenital rubella are extremely important. The child may be mentally retarded and deaf, so early recognition of ocular problems and their treatment are vital. The treatable defects include cataract, glaucoma, squint and refractive errors. The cataract may not appear until several weeks or months after birth, so the eyes should be re-examined. There may be a diffuse retinopathy ("salt and pepper" appearance).

Acquired immune deficiency syndrome (AIDS)

The ocular complications of AIDS can be blinding. Manifestations include Kaposi's sarcoma of the conjunctiva, retinal haemorrhages and vasculitis. Cotton wool spots may appear and disappear spontaneously, and their presence signifies a poor prognosis even in a patient without symptoms. Ocular cytomegalovirus infection presents as areas of retinal opacification with haemorrhages and exudates that proceed to severe ocular damage, including retinal detachment.

Various antiviral agents, however, have proved useful in the treatment of ocular complications, but may have to be taken continuously, and systemic side effects from these treatments are not uncommon. Intraocular implants that release local antiviral agents reduce systemic complications. Blindness resulting from the ocular complications of AIDS used to be one of the major reasons for suicide in AIDS patients. Fortunately, new drugs, particularly the protease inhibitors, have dramatically reduced the incidence of ocular cytomegalovirus infection.

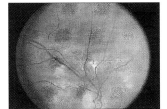

Cytomegalovirus retinitis in AIDS.

12 The eye and the nervous system

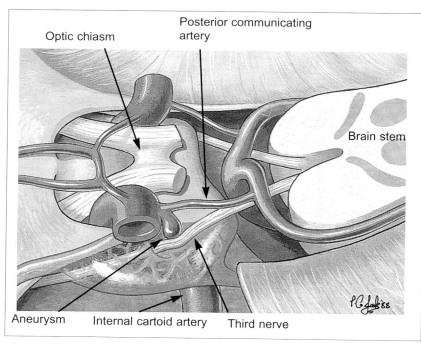

Optic chiasm

Posterior communicating artery

Brain stem

Aneurysm   Internal cartoid artery   Third nerve

Posterior communicating artery aneurysm compressing third nerve.

Nerves of eye movement

Ocular signs may be the first indication of serious neurological disease. Alternatively, the eyes may be responsible for "neurological" symptoms such as headache.

Palsies of the third, fourth and sixth cranial nerves all cause paralytic squints in which the angle of squint varies with the direction of gaze. Adult patients may also complain of double vision, so it is important to exclude palsies of these three nerves when examining patients who have either a squint or double vision.

Third nerve palsy — A patient with a third nerve palsy may present with a variety of symptoms depending on the cause of the palsy. He may complain of a drooping eyelid, double vision (if the lid does not cover the eye), or headache in the distribution of the ophthalmic division of the trigeminal nerve.

On examination there is characteristically a ptosis (paralysed levator muscle of the eyelid) and the eye is turned out because of the action of the unaffected lateral rectus muscle that is supplied by the sixth nerve. The eye is sometimes turned slightly downwards because of the unopposed action of the unaffected superior oblique muscle supplied by the fourth nerve. The pupil is dilated because the parasympathetic fibres of the third nerve supplying the sphincter pupillae are damaged.

Important causes of a third nerve palsy include intracranial aneurysms, compressive lesions in the cavernous sinus and diabetes. The presence of pain and a dilated pupil mean that a compressive lesion must be excluded urgently, as treatment may be life saving and curative for what may be an otherwise fatal lesion such as an aneurysm.

Fourth nerve palsy — This is often difficult to diagnose. There may be a compensatory head tilt in that the head will be tilted away from the side of the lesion and the chin will be depressed. The fourth nerve is long and is therefore particularly susceptible to injury. A patient with bilateral fourth nerve palsies following a head injury may complain only of difficulty in reading. This occurs as a result of difficulty during depression and convergence of the eyes because both superior oblique muscles are paralysed. This diagnosis should be considered in any patient who complains of difficulty in reading after a head injury.

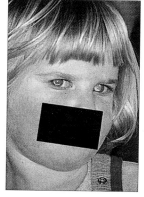

Abnormal head posture in right fourth nerve palsy.

Sixth nerve palsy — This is probably the best known of the palsies of the three nerves of ocular motility. The eye on the affected side cannot be abducted. The patient develops horizontal diplopia that worsens when he looks towards the side of the affected muscle. It is important to recognize a sixth nerve palsy, as it may be the result of raised intracranial pressure that is causing compression of the nerve.

Management
This is initially directed to making an accurate diagnosis. If diplopia is a problem, opaque sticky tape may be placed over the patient's glasses, or a patch may be placed over the eye. Adults will not develop amblyopia. Temporary prisms may be put on the glasses if the angle is not too large. For long term treatment, permanent prisms (which are clearer than temporary prisms) may be incorporated into a prescription for spectacles. Later, an operation may be performed to straighten the eyes.

Facial nerve palsy

Seventh nerve palsy
Facial weakness caused by a seventh nerve palsy is common. In many cases no cause is found and the palsy improves spontaneously. If the eyelids do not close properly corneal exposure, ulceration, and eventual scarring and blindness may occur. Ocular assessment should include:

Testing of corneal sensation — The cornea is innervated by the ophthalmic branch of the fifth nerve, which may also be affected by the pathology that is causing the seventh nerve palsy.. If the corneal sensation is impaired the patient should be referred to an ophthalmic surgeon, as there is a high risk of corneal scarring. Patients cannot feel foreign bodies or feel when their corneas are ulcerating. In such a case this is in addition to being unable to close the eye and lubricate the cornea.

Testing of Bell's phenomenon (not to be confused with a Bell's palsy) — Normally when the eyes are closed the eyes move up under the upper lids. This "Bell's phenomenon" can be tested by asking the patient with a facial palsy to close his eyes while the observer watches the position of the cornea. If the cornea does not move up under the paralysed lid the patient is at a high risk of developing corneal exposure.

Staining the cornea with fluorescein — If there is staining of the cornea when fluorescein is used this indicates the cornea is drying out. If there is only a tiny amount of stain, the eye is white and quiet, and the visual acuity is normal the patient may be managed in the short term with tear drops and ointment. If the staining persists or if the eye becomes red then he should be referred straight away to an ophthalmologist. The cornea may need to be protected by frequent lubrication and possibly sewing together the lateral parts of the eyelids or lowering the upper eyelid with botulinum toxin.

Sympathetic pathway

Horner's syndrome
In a patient with Horner's syndrome the sympathetic nerve supply to the eye is disturbed. The clinical features are:

A small pupil that is reactive to light (unlike the small pupil caused by pilocarpine eye drops) because the sympathetically innervated dilator muscle of the pupil are paralysed.

A drooping eyelid — The muscles that raise the eyelid are innervated by the third nerve and also by the sympathetic nerve supply. Therefore lesions of either the third nerve or the sympathetic nervous system supplying these muscles cause a ptosis, though in the latter case it is only slight.

Management of paralytic squint.

- Diagnosis
- Patch
- Temporary prism
- Permanent prism
- ? Operation

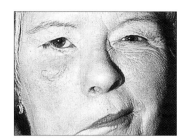
Right facial palsy. The eyelids on the right have been partly sewn together to protect the eye.

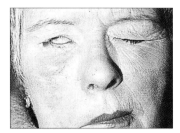
Cornea moves up under upper lid on attempted closure of the eye.

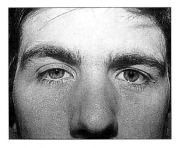
Right Horner's syndrome.

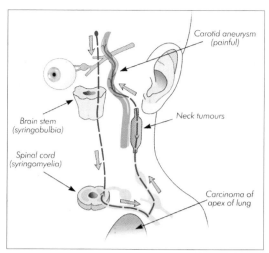

Sites of lesions of the sympathetic pathway to the eye.

Lack of sweating on the same side of the face is again because of sympathetic denervation and depends on the position of the lesion. The ocular movements are completely normal as the extraocular muscles are not sympathetically innervated. The figure shows the pathway of the sympathetic system and the possible causes of Horner's syndrome.

Optic disc

The swollen optic disc

There are many causes of a swollen optic disc, the best known of which is raised intracranial pressure resulting in the development of papilloedema. The absence of papilloedema, however, does not exclude raised intracranial pressure. It is the history and examination of the patient that should lead to the suspicion of raised intracranial pressure, and a swollen optic disc is merely a helpful sign. The vision of patients with papilloedema is usually not affected until late in the course of the disease. Most causes of a swollen disc are serious from either the ocular or systemic point of view, and patients should be referred promptly. If a patient has a swollen optic disc the following features suggest a diagnosis other than raised intracranial pressure.

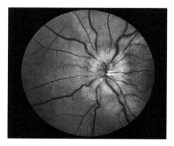

Papilloedema: swollen disc secondary to raised intraocular pressure.

Impaired vision — Vision is usually impaired only late in the course of papilloedema. It is crucial to consider giant cell arteritis in the presence of impaired vision and the patient may or may not have, in addition, aching muscles, malaise, headaches, tenderness over the temporal arteries, and claudication of the jaw muscles when eating. The disc is characteristically swollen and pale because the small vessels that supply the head of the optic nerve are inflamed and occluded. By this time the vision will be severely affected. **It is important to exclude giant cell arteritis in any patient over 60 with visual disturbance or a swollen optic disc** as urgent treatment with steroids should be instituted to prevent blindness in the other eye.

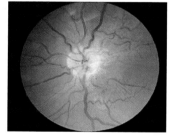

Optic nerurits.

Disturbance of the visual fields — The visual fields of a patient with raised intracranial pressure are usually normal. The presence of a field defect should lead one to suspect some other diagnosis such as compression of the optic nerve.

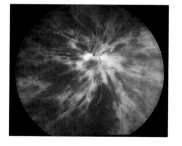

Swollen disc secondary to central retinal vein occlusion.

A pale disc — The disc of a patient with raised intracranial pressure is often hyperaemic. It is only in longstanding papilloedema that the disc becomes atrophic and pale. The disc is also pale if the swelling results from ischaemia of the optic nerve, as in giant cell arteritis.

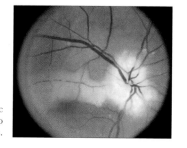

Swollen disc secondary to temporal arteritis.

Retinal exudates and haemorrhages — These are present in papilloedema and are usually found around the disc. If there are many exudates or haemorrhages in the retina diagnoses such as retinal vein occlusion, malignant hypertension, diabetes, and vasculitis should be considered. In all patients the blood pressure should be measured and the urine tested for the presence of sugar, blood, and protein.

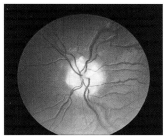

Optic nerve head drusen.

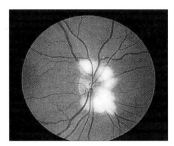

Myelinated nerve fibres.

"Headache" around the eye: important features.

- Nature of pain
- Associated visual disturbance
- Red eye
- Defective ocular movements
- Abnormal pupils
- Abnormal optic disc

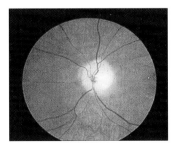

Optic atrophy.

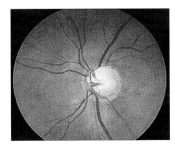

Glaucomatous cupping.

Conditions that may mimic swelling of the head of the optic nerve include:

- *Longsightedness* (hypermetropia), in which the margin of the optic disc does not look clear. A clue lies in the patient's glasses, which make the patients eyes look larger.
- *Drusen of the head of the optic nerve* — These colloid bodies of the head of the nerve makes the margin of the disc look blurred.
- *Developmental abnormalities of the head of the nerve* — These may be difficult to diagnose.

The pale optic disc

There are many causes of a pale optic disc and it is important to make the correct diagnosis as many of them are treatable. These include compressive lesions, glaucoma, vitamin deficiency, the presence of toxic substances (for example, lead or some drugs) and infective conditions such as syphilis. It is also important to identify whether the cause is hereditary as genetic counselling, and occasionally, metabolic treatments are available (for example, a diet free of phytanic acid and plasma exchange may prevent the progression of ocular disease in Refsum's disease).

Headaches and the eye

Most patients who present with a history of "headache" around the eye do not have serious disease. Points in the history and examination that should raise suspicion of serious disease include:

The nature of the headache — Headaches that cause sleep disturbance, or that are worse on waking or with coughing, suggest raised intracranial pressure. Temporal tenderness in patients over the age of 60 with symptoms of aching muscles and malaise suggest giant cell arteritis.

Visual disturbance — If there is a change in visual acuity that cannot be corrected by a pinhole test, serious disease should be suspected. A history of haloes around lights (caused by transient oedema of the cornea when the intraocular pressure rises) suggests attacks of angle closure glaucoma.

A red eye — In acute glaucoma the eye is usually red, injected and tender, and the acuity is diminished. The pain is deep seated and may be associated with vomiting. Inflammation of the iris and ciliary body also cause a red eye and a deep pain. Primary open angle glaucoma does not present with severe pain.

Defective ocular movements — If there are restricted ocular movements on the same side as the pain, serious disease must be suspected. This may include orbital cellulitis (from infected sinuses), inflammatory lesions in the orbit, and compressive lesions causing nerve palsies (for example, a posterior communicating aneurysm causing third nerve palsy and pain around the eye).

Abnormal pupils — An abnormal pupil on the side of the headache should suggest a compressive lesion (for example, a painful Horner's syndrome caused by an internal carotid aneurysm).

In so called "cluster headaches" and "ophthalmoplegic migraine" pupillary abnormalities and ocular motility problems may be present in these relatively benign conditions. Patients with headache around the eye, however, together with ocular motility or pupillary abnormalities, should be investigated to exclude serious lesions.

Swelling, atrophy, or cupping of the optic disc — If a patient with headaches around the eye has any of these findings referral is required. The swelling and atrophy may be due to a compressive lesion and pathological cupping suggests a chronic form of glaucoma.

Index

Page numbers in **bold** type refer to figures; those in *italic* refer to tables or boxed material.